SpringerBriefs in Applied Sciences and Technology

Computational Intelligence

Series editor

Janusz Kacprzyk, Polish Academy of Sciences, Systems Research Institute, Warsaw, Poland

The series "Studies in Computational Intelligence" (SCI) publishes new developments and advances in the various areas of computational intelligence—quickly and with a high quality. The intent is to cover the theory, applications, and design methods of computational intelligence, as embedded in the fields of engineering, computer science, physics and life sciences, as well as the methodologies behind them. The series contains monographs, lecture notes and edited volumes in computational intelligence spanning the areas of neural networks, connectionist systems, genetic algorithms, evolutionary computation, artificial intelligence, cellular automata, self-organizing systems, soft computing, fuzzy systems, and hybrid intelligent systems. Of particular value to both the contributors and the readership are the short publication timeframe and the world-wide distribution, which enable both wide and rapid dissemination of research output.

More information about this series at http://www.springer.com/series/10618

Gita Khalili Moghaddam
Christopher R. Lowe

Health and Wellness Measurement Approaches for Mobile Healthcare

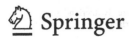 Springer

Gita Khalili Moghaddam
Department of Pharmacology
University of Cambridge
Cambridge, UK

and

Department of Chemical Engineering
and Biotechnology
University of Cambridge
Cambridge, UK

Christopher R. Lowe
Department of Pharmacology
University of Cambridge
Cambridge, UK

and

Department of Chemical Engineering
and Biotechnology
University of Cambridge
Cambridge, UK

ISSN 2191-530X   ISSN 2191-5318   (electronic)
SpringerBriefs in Applied Sciences and Technology
ISSN 2625-3704   ISSN 2625-3712   (electronic)
SpringerBriefs in Computational Intelligence
ISBN 978-3-030-01556-5   ISBN 978-3-030-01557-2   (eBook)
https://doi.org/10.1007/978-3-030-01557-2

Library of Congress Control Number: 2018956269

This Springer imprint is published by the registered company Springer Nature Switzerland AG
The registered company address is: Gewerbestrasse 11, 6330 Cham, Switzerland

Acknowledgements

The authors would like to express their gratitude to the University of Cambridge for providing the opportunity to publish this book. We also would like to offer our appreciation to all those individuals who provided help in publication of this book.

Contents

Abbreviations

2G	Second generation of communication technology
3D	Three-dimensional
4G	Fourth generation of communication technology
A/D	Analog-to-digital
Apps	Mobile applications
ASD	Autism spectrum disorder
BAN	Body area network
BCG	Ballistocardiogram
BMI	Body mass Index
bps	Bits per second
CAD	Coronary artery disease
CAGR	Compound annual growth rate
CE	Conformité Européene—European Conformity
CIN	Cervical intraepithelial neoplasia
COPD	Chronic obstructive pulmonary disorder
CVD	Cardiovascular diseases
D	Diopter—a unit measuring a lens' refractive power
DALYs	Disability-adjusted life years
DLW	Doubly labeled water
DR	Diabetic retinopathy
ECG	Electrocardiogram
EEG	Electroencephalogram
EMG	Electromyogram
FDA	Food and Drug Administration
FEV1	Forced expiratory volume in one second
FOG	Freeze of Gait
FuzzyEn	Fuzzy entropy
FVC	Forced vital capacity
GDP	Gross domestic product
GPS	Global Positioning System

HRV	Heart rate variability
Hz	Hertz
iPPG	Imaging photoplethysmogram
IR	Infrared
ISDN	Integrated Services for Digital Networks
LCD	Liquid crystal Display
LED	Light-emitting diode
LMICs	Lower-middle-income Countries
LWIR	Long-wavelength infrared
MET	Metabolic equivalent
mhealth	Mobile healthcare
OS	Operating system
PAEE	Physical activity energy expenditure
PD	Parkinson's disease
PEF	Peak expiratory flow
PPG	Photoplethysmogram
qEEG	Quantitative electroencephalogram
REE	Resting energy expenditure
RGB	Red–green–blue
ROI	Region of interest
RR	Relative risks
SampEn	Sample entropy
sEMG	Surface electromyogram
SMS	Short message services
SO_2	Arterial oxygen saturation
T2DM	Type 2 diabetes mellitus
TEE	Total energy expenditure
TEF	Thermic effect of food
VIA	Visual inspection with 4% (v/v) acetic acid
WHO	World Health Organization

Chapter 1
Mobile Healthcare

1.1 Current Healthcare Challenges

There is a substantial body of research pointing to numerous challenges in the current provision of healthcare (Fig. 1.1). The principal issue is rising healthcare expenditure, which is primarily posed by global and demographic changes, such as economic growth and urbanisation. The Gross Domestic Product (GDP) value has a positive impact on the average human lifespan, whereas urbanisation has a negative impact on health. The total dependency ratio (the ratio of non-working age to working age for the population) is expected to rise sharply as a result of a continued increase in human longevity. For instance, the ratio in Japan, North America, Western Europe and China will reach 73.8, 33, 44 and 38%, respectively, while the global average ratio will be 25% in 2050 [1]. In terms of health status, the influence of modernisation on lifestyle and dietary habits, such as the tendency of eating processed food, is linked to the prevalence of chronic diseases such as Type 2 Diabetes Mellitus (T2DM), Chronic Obstructive Pulmonary Disorder (COPD), cardiovascular diseases (CVD) and cancer. By 2035, for example, it is expected that the prevalence of T2DM in the EU will be 70M [2].

Managing the combination of chronic diseases and an ageing population is leading to unsustainable healthcare costs and rising morbidity. Healthcare costs in the US, European countries and China reached 17.9, 8–9 and 4.5% of GDP in 2010, respectively [3], implying that the *per capita* healthcare expenditure has grown faster than income levels and inflation [4]. The underlying cause of increasing costs is that the current healthcare model behaves in a reactive manner and is episodic in nature and thus, is not often suitable to manage patients who are routinely flagged for treatment once their condition has deteriorated to a point where significant morbidity and complications develop. A preferred approach is, therefore, frequent and/or real-time monitoring of patients, which can offer a means to anticipate an increased risk of failing health and thus act upon the warning signs at an earlier stage and eventually reduce hospital admissions for acute treatment. While this approach may lower

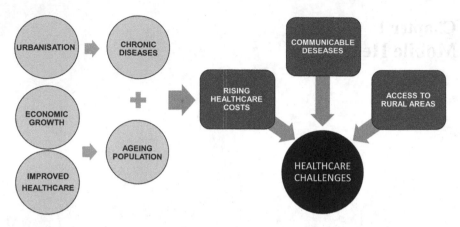

Fig. 1.1 Current healthcare challenges

healthcare costs, there are two overarching concerns associated with this strategy, i.e. the growing trend towards professional outsourcing and the resultant labour hours lost. In response to these issues, healthcare organisations are looking at a *patient-centred* model to empower patients to manage their conditions at homes or wherever they happen to be, but outside high-cost healthcare institutions such as hospitals and surgeries.

While the prevalence of chronic diseases and ageing are raising the burden on healthcare systems across the world, developing countries are dealing with two additional challenges. One is the elimination of communicable diseases: In developing countries, communicable diseases are the leading cause of mortality, 36%, while accounting for 40% of total annual DALYs (Disability Adjusted Life Years) lost [5]. The underlying health-related causes of communicable diseases are the absence of knowledge of appropriate health countermeasures, lack of access to public sources of medical knowledge, shortage of high-level health professionals and inadequate health education programs to train health educators. Therefore, efforts to address communicable diseases need to focus on disseminating relevant health information and strengthening healthcare surveillance at the local, national and global levels. Another additional challenge of developing nations is extending healthcare access in rural areas. Developing countries are predominantly rural (68.5% in 2010 and 66.3% in 2015 [6]) and are characterised by a shortage of financial resources to support both the physical infrastructure of healthcare and professionals. To cope with the challenges of rural healthcare, the healthcare system should aim at empowering lower-level health personnel in remote communities by linking them to higher-level ones in the urban areas to obtain peer advice, thereby enabling evidence-based diagnosis by using cost-effective diagnostic instruments and, at the same time, providing geographically remote consultation with specialists for patients.

These major challenges are exacerbated by the emerging expectations of healthcare stakeholders. From the demand perspective, individuals press for timely access to high-quality personalised healthcare services anywhere at any time, namely *the third place* [3], in a trusted way. On the supply side, a shift from a *sick-care* to a *health-care* model is expected, where the focus of the former is diagnosis and treatment and that of the latter is wellness and prevention. This transformation entails activating responsible citizens to take more informed decisions on their health.

1.2 Mobile Healthcare (mHealth)

To tackle the challenges being imposed on the healthcare industry, healthcare organisations are looking at *value* as a solution strategy. Value in healthcare systems is a function of favourable outcomes and healthcare costs:

$$\text{Value} = \frac{\text{Outcomes}}{\text{Costs}} \tag{1.1}$$

where the health outcomes encompass timely access, service quality, equity, affordability, quality of life and the overall national health status [7], while variables contributing to healthcare costs include the number of patients, the number of visits, the number and type of services per episode of care and costs per service (Fig. 1.2) [8]. Given the low cost, immediacy and widespread availability of mobile technology (Sect. 1.3), healthcare experts agree that the integration of mobile technology with existing healthcare settings appears to have the potential to maximise the value proposition for healthcare. The deployment of a mobile-enabled healthcare (mhealth) model can leverage the capacity and quality of health services by sharing accountability and responsibility between healthcare consumers and suppliers. In this healthcare system, the focus is on prevention by enabling self-management and, if care is needed, it is based on evidence, informed patient preferences and shared decisions. Additionally, mhealth services can improve health outcomes by the arrival of healthcare everywhere, transparency in pricing, convenience in routine testing and efficiency of treatment. Moreover, mhealth can reduce healthcare costs over time and thus offer a financially sustainable system. For instance, promoting healthy behaviour and prevention using mhealth interventions can reduce the number of patients, while mhealth enables remote monitoring of patients and thus reduces the number of outpatient follow-up visits. Accordingly, mhealth can potentially create a broad socio-economic impact for the various beneficiaries.

The architecture of an mhealth ecosystem integrates three key components: A Body Area Network (BAN), a cloud-based server and healthcare providers (Fig. 1.3), where a BAN is a subset of a sensor network (body gateway) and a host device. Nodes in the body gateway are capable of generating sensory information using a combination of on- and off-body, embedded and ambient sensors. On-body sensors refer to wearable sensors and intelligent clothes and off-body sensors are home, workplace and point-of-care diagnostics tests. Every sensor node has a wired/wireless communication module to establish a secure connection with the cloud server through a host

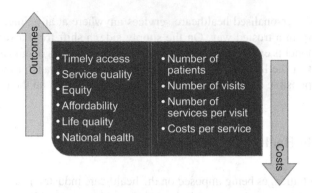

Fig. 1.2 Potential of mhealth in improving healthcare outcomes and reducing healthcare expenditure

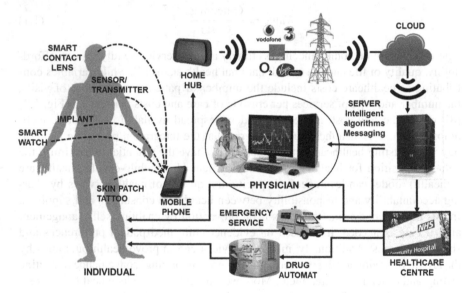

Fig. 1.3 The mHealth system architecture

device to transfer data from and to the patient remote site. Besides data gathering, aggregation and dissemination, the host device performs other key tasks: Preliminary data processing, data visualisation and local data storage. The advanced data analysis and big data storage capabilities offered by cloud services allow healthcare centres to gain data literacy and provide the required health information to the user, medical professionals and payers.

To provide a historical perspective and technical background on the concept of mhealth, the first following section reviews mobile technology by presenting the evolution of mobile technology, value-added mobile features and its business implication and emerging trends. Then, new horizons for health through mobile technology, the process of implementing mobile technology into the healthcare industry and challenges are thoroughly described.

1.3 Mobile Technology

Mobile technology has unique features not available to traditional wired electronic technologies and is revolutionising both our society and the business world. Mobile technology offers a novel mode of liberty for individuals: "free, yet tracked; mobile, yet contained" [9]. In this respect, mobile technology presents a new mode of business transaction which promises many alluring market opportunities.

1.3.1 Overview of Mobile Technology

The mobile phone presents itself as something that followed the trajectory of the telephone, and then telecommunications. However, very quickly, mobile phones have established themselves as a central culture in their own right, and tend towards an emphasis on constant contact with the individual rather than the household as well as qualities of mobility, portability and customisation. With continually rising expectations about mobility and a widening access to wireless connectivity, mobile technology has taken a turn forward and picked up significant speed since the first mobile phone was introduced in 1979 [10]. The evolution of mobile technology has to a large extent been spawned by technological advances in both mobile networks and mobile phone handsets.

1.3.1.1 Mobile Networks

The mobile network is one platform involved in enabling mobile technology. Mobile networks are commonly divided into generations: The first mobile network generation (1G) was analogue and only supported voice transmission. As demand grew, the second generation (2G) of communication technology was developed in 1991. This generation was a type of Integrated Services for Digital Networks (ISDN) and therefore supported both voice and data, while it enhanced the number of services for global evolutions such as text messages, picture messages and multi-media messages (MMS). Later in the 1990s, the operators of 2G systems offered more efficient forms of data transmission, known as 2.5G and 2.75G, to enhance the speed of data transmission from 56 to 153.6 Kbps. In 2001, so-called 3G networks were commercially launched, which not only enabled the worldwide use of services such as web browsing, metre accuracy GPS (Global Positioning System) and multimedia services, but also provided better bandwidth and higher data transmission rates, up to 2 Mbps [10]. Currently, 4G is available in networks around the world and has enabled mobile ultra-broadband internet access to support data-transmission speeds as high as, and in excess of, 100 Mbps. According to the International Telecommunication Union specifications in 2015, 5G networks are expected to be deployed by 2020, which will support up to 1 Tbps, with the promise of an enhanced quality of service.

1.3.1.2   Mobile Phones

It is not just mobile network technology that makes mobile communication possible; users need personal devices to access the mobile network through mobile terminals. Since the technology incorporated into mobile handsets has a significant impact on services that can be offered, their development was another fundamental brick in the emergence of advanced mobile technology.

When mobile networks first began, there was a basic model of mobile phone available to support only voice. Basic mobile phones offered a simple model with a monochrome screen and single-tasking environment, and were often bulky and had poor battery lives. Advances in all aspects of mobile phone technology during the 1980s meant that handsets became smaller and battery life improved. These internet-enabled handsets, so-called feature phones, incorporated advanced features such as megapixel cameras, video capture, Bluetooth, expandable memory slots, and Java capability. By the late 1990s, smartphones started to enter the marketplace at a fast pace. The smartphone is generally defined as a hybrid device whose primary function is that of a phone, communication, with added advanced computing capabilities with a low-power Operating System (OS). Meanwhile, high-quality graphical interfaces have provided a platform to introduce virtual keyboards and sophisticated touchscreen capability. The design of smartphones also relies on the use of embedded sensors to optimise the platform operation and to offer higher level services to the users. Embedded sensors (Fig. 1.4) in handsets include motion detectors (for measuring acceleration and rotational forces), environmental sensors (for measuring temperature, illumination, pressure, humidity), position sensors (for measuring orientation and magnetic North), sound sensors (for sound processing) and CMOS image sensors (for capturing image, colour analysis and pattern recognition).

Alongside the hardware innovations, new software architectures have been created to support the device hardware features, which are referred to as mobile applications (apps). Smartphone users can download apps through app stores using built-in Wi-Fi features to perform specific functions in various sectors such as agriculture, education, financial services, social networking, information services, gaming and health. In terms of development and implementation, it is possible to run apps on mobile devices, *native apps*, and or remotely in the cloud, *cloud apps*.

Native apps invade the mobile space and rely on its restricted computational power while anchoring users to a proprietary OS (Google Android, iOS, Microsoft and Symbian), whereas cloud apps can be used independently of the OS, albeit using a mobile broadband subscription. Another benefit arising from cloud computing

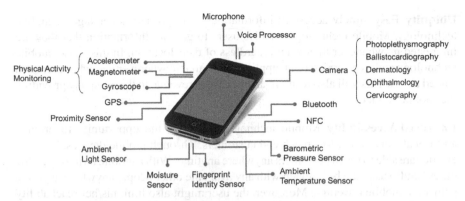

Fig. 1.4 Embedded sensors in smartphones and their potential application in healthcare (*Source for the smartphone image* Adapted from [11])

is that less mobile space and computational power on the phone are required; the latter is related to lower power consumption and thus saving battery life. In this context, the cloud-computing strategy has the potential to leverage an infrastructure to perform computationally expensive tasks such as digital image/sound processing and therefore holds opportunities for app development in new domains. Despite the advantages of cloud apps over native apps, a compelling argument is that most embedded sensors are not accessible via cloud apps. However, cloud apps are gaining access to more built-in sensors as the technology progresses.

The interaction between apps and sensors has transformed smartphones to affordable and easy-to-use measuring tools and will continue to incorporate more innovative functionality in the following years by interacting with developments in a diverse range of vertical sectors such as healthcare. The list of sensors that apps in the healthcare sector can interact with is going beyond solely embedded phone sensors. Emerging apps, namely *sensor apps*, work in conjunction with external peripheral sensors. Auxiliary sensors, including a wide range of sensors from implantable to wearable to portable sensors, measure quantities (vital signs, chemicals and metabolites) and then interface with embedded sensors (e.g. Bluetooth and optical) to transfer raw data to sensor apps for visualization, recording, preliminary/advanced processing and transferring to a predefined cloud.

1.3.2 Features of Mobile Technology

The essence of mobile technology is about providing the technological infrastructure for maintaining easy access to information at the right time regardless of where users are with minimal upfront expenditure [12]. Accordingly, mobile technology is associated with a set of value-added features:

Ubiquity Easy, timely access to information is the primary advantage of mobile technology. Mobile technology enables users to get any information that they are interested in, whenever they want regardless of their location. In this sense, mobile technology makes a service or an application available wherever and whenever such a need arises. This will also result in an increase in revenue to the company providing the mobile services.

Improved Accessibility Mobile technology presents the opportunity to provide additional value to hard-to-reach end customers. Through mobile devices, business entities are able to reach customers anywhere anytime. With a mobile terminal, on the other hand, a user can be in touch with any available other people anywhere anytime, subject to mobile coverage. Moreover, the user might also limit his/her reachability to a particular person or at particular times.

Localisation The knowledge of the user's physical location at a particular moment also adds significant value to mobile technology. With location information available, many location-based services (LBS) can be provided including emergency caller location, navigation, and geographically targeted advertisements.

Personalisation Given the enormous number of services and apps that are currently available in the app market, the mobile ecosystem can be explicitly adapted based on the preference of the user to represent information and provide services in a way appropriate to the user.

Feedback Loop Mobile technology has the ability to collect objective data from users, share them and provide insight and goals which can be achieved through personalised choices.

Dissemination Some wireless infrastructures support simultaneous delivery of data to all mobile users within a specific geographical region. This functionality offers an efficient means to disseminate information to a large consumer population.

1.3.3   Business Implications of Mobile Technology

According to the latest annual report from ITU, the United Nations agency responsible for looking into the world's Information and Communication Technology issues, there would be 6.8B mobile subscriptions by the end of 2013, taking global mobile penetration to close to 100%. The massive growth of adoption and advancement of mobile technology creates opportunities for providing a range of innovative mobile services through mobile apps. The market for mobile apps was launched by the Apple App Store in 2008 and, after its immediate success, app stores of other OS providers emerged. In two years, the apps market reached 10B app downloads with a global revenue of US$2.2B, demonstrating a 160.2% increase. In 2017, global app downloads from both App Store and Google Play reached 175B where users spent

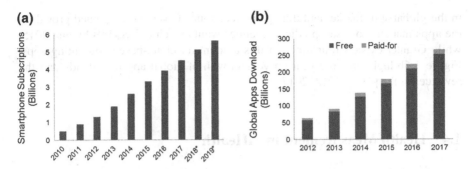

Fig. 1.5 a Global smartphone penetration, 2010–2019* (Adopted from [14]). *Note* *Estimate, **b** download of mobile apps from all stores worldwide, 2012–2017* (Adopted from [15])

US$58.6B on apps, including in-app purchases, subscriptions and premium apps [13].

The most important trend underpinning the fast pace of growth of the apps market is global smartphone penetration, although there are differences in the estimated growth rate. For example, according to Ericsson [14], global smartphone subscriptions will amount to 5.6B, or 60% of the total mobile subscriptions, by the end of 2019, compared to 1.9 billion in 2013, or 30% of the total mobile subscriptions (Fig. 1.5a). This growth will be led by markets in Africa and Eastern Europe, followed by the Middle East, Latin America, and Asia-Pacific, while the advanced markets of Western Europe and North America are approaching saturation [16]. The first and foremost driving factor in the global spread of smartphones is the rapid fall in their price, particularly in emerging markets [17]. Today, smartphone users usually come from top-earning socioeconomic groups; however, with various factors (local subsidies, domestic manufacture, high-level competition) combining to lowering smartphone prices, smartphones are expected to become accessible to a greater proportion of the world population. According to the International Data Corporation the average global price of a smartphone, which was US$368 in 2013, fell to US$303 in 2017 [18].

Another trend that is driving the increased download of mobile apps is the growth of mobile-broadband subscriptions which provides access to bandwidth-intense value-added services. Mobile-broadband subscriptions are estimated to reach 6.5B by 2018 [19]. It should be noted that mathematical models predict a substantial difference in average annual growth (CAGR) of mobile broadband subscription (2007–2017) in developed and developing regions, with 18% in the former compared with 38% in the latter. The predicted upsurge in mobile-broadband subscriptions in developing countries is primarily driven by the lack of infrastructure for deployment of the fixed (wired)-broadband, particularly in rural areas. Rural inhabitants of developing countries account for 66.3% in 2015 [6] of the population. Given the infrastructure challenge to provide fixed-broadband services for these people, mobile-broadband, which is less complicated to deploy, is considered an alternative. Accordingly, developing countries are playing an increasingly important role in the global apps market and thus global economy. Given the continued growth in the apps market, Forrester predicts revenues would reach to US$38B by end 2015, while Granter expects four times of this amount for cloud-based computing apps. Figure 1.5b highlights the year-on-year growth of global app downloads and the revenue for the period 2012–2017.

1.4 Health Measurement in mHealth

The concept of health is overarching and the index of health status includes a complex set of physical, physiological, psychological, subjective and social indicators. Accordingly, defining a set of standard criteria to fulfil the broad definition of health and incorporate various levels of complexity and the relationships among them is challenging [20–23]. In line with the framework of this book, a choice of indicators on different aspects of health status that can be remotely monitored is considered. For each health indicator, the capacity of sensor technologies to be applicable to mhealth and the likely clinical outcomes are explored in depth in two sections of physical activity and ex vivo biosignatures in following chapters.

References

1. PwC (2012) Touching lives through mobile health: assessment of the global Market opportunity
2. European Coalition for Diabetes (2014) Diabetes in europe. Policy Puzzle, The state we are in
3. Ernst & Young E (2012) Mobile technology poised to enable new era in health care
4. The World Bank (2016) Health nutrition and population statistics
5. Skolnik R (2008) Essentials of global health. Jones & Bartlett Learning, USA
6. Department of Economic and Social Affairs, UN (2013) Urban and rural population by age and sex, 1980–2015
7. Adams J, Bakalar R, Boroch M, Knecht K, Mounib EL, Stuart N (2013) Healthcare 2015 and care delivery: delivery models refined, competencies define. IBM Global Business Services
8. Scheel O, Anscombe J, Wintermantel T, Reincke E (2013) Mobile health: mirage or growth opportunity? A. T. Kearney Korea LLC
9. May P (2001) Mobile commerce: opportunities, applications, and technologies of wireless business. Cambridge University Press, UK
10. Wakefield T, McNally D, Bowler D, Mayne A (2012) Introduction to mobile communications: technology, services, markets: technology, services, markets. Taylor & Francis, UK
11. Zanetti D Iphone 4. Wikipedia. https://de.wikipedia.org/wiki/Datei:Iphone_4G-3_grey_scree n.png#/media/File:Iphone_4G-3_grey_screen.png. Accessed Feb 2018
12. Siau K, Lim E-P, Shen Z (2001) Mobile commerce: promises, challenges and research agenda. J Database Manag 12(3):4–13
13. Nelson R (2018) Global app revenue grew 35% in 2017 to nearly $60 billion SensorTower Inc. https://sensortower.com/blog/app-revenue-and-downloads-2017. Accessed Feb 2018
14. Ericsson (2013) Ericsson mobility report: global smartphone subscriptions to reach 5.6 billion by 2019
15. Gartner (2013) Gartner says free apps will account for nearly 90 percent of total mobile app store downloads in 2012. http://www.gartner.com/newsroom/id/2592315. Accessed Jan 2018

16. Portio Research (2013) Portio research mobile factbook 2013
17. Lemaitre G (2012) The smartphone boom in emerging markets. http://www.gfk-geomarket ing.com/en/about_geomarketing/gfk_geomarketing_magazine/012013/the_smartphone_boo m_in_emerging_markets.html. Accessed Apr 2016
18. International Data Corporation (2013) IDC finds worldwide smartphone shipments on pace to grow nearly 40% in 2013 while average selling prices decline more than 12% business wire. https://www.businesswire.com/news/home/20131126005293/en/IDC-Finds-World wide-Smartphone-Shipments-Pace-Grow. Accessed May 2016
19. International Telecommunication Union (2013) Measuring the information society 2013
20. Jenkinson C, McGee HM (1998) Health status measurement: a brief but critical introduction. Radcliffe Medical Press, UK
21. McDowell I (2006) Measuring health: a guide to rating scales and questionnaires. Oxford University Press, UK
22. Kaplan RM, Bush JW, Berry CC (1976) Health status: types of validity and the index of well-being. Health Serv Res 11(4):478–507
23. OECD (2011) How's life? measuring well-being: measuring well-being. OECD Publishing, France

Chapter 2
Physical Activity

2.1 Introduction

The correlation between sedentary lifestyles and health consequences such as overweight (Body Mass Index (BMI) of 25–29.9) and obesity (BMI > 30) [1–5], diabetes mellitus (DM) [6–8], cardiovascular diseases (CVD) [9–11] and cancer [12] is clinically proven [13]. According to the WHO [14], sedentary lifestyles with a prevalence of 23% in adults (>18 years) accounts for 6% of global mortality. The total economic burden of a sedentary lifestyle in the US in 2003 was ~US$251B [15]. Physical activity also plays a critical role in achieving a greater level of life quality and independence [16]. Therefore, it is desirable to develop an automated lifestyle intervention paradigm which will boost awareness and incentivise changes in physical behaviour.

Before one considers the implementation of such interventions to promote physical activity, it is necessary to understand the key concepts behind this paradigm: Physical activity, models of conceptualising physical activity and the assessment and quantitation of the level of physical activity. According to the Department of Health and Human Services [17], physical activity is "any bodily movement produced by skeletal muscles that result in increased energy expenditure above a basal level (resting level)". Physical activity can occur in four broad domains including occupational (labour task, carrying objects), domestic (housework, gardening, child care, chores), transportation (walking, cycling, standing), and leisure time (sport, exercise, hobbies) [18]. Conventional approaches promote physical activity with a focus primarily on the leisure time domain. However, the substitution effect of physical activity and hence the health benefits from all four domains of physical activity have been identified in cohort studies [19]. This necessitates monitoring of the total physical activity during daily life to obtain habitual activity levels. Furthermore, it is important to identify the relative time spent in each of the physical activity dimensions.

G. Khalili Moghaddam and C. R. Lowe, *Health and Wellness Measurement Approaches for Mobile Healthcare*, SpringerBriefs in Computational Intelligence, https://doi.org/10.1007/978-3-030-01557-2_2

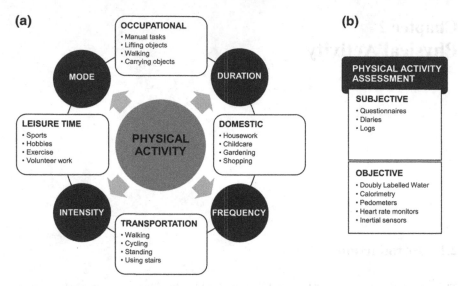

Fig. 2.1 **a** Physical activity domains and dimensions, **b** physical activity assessment methods

As shown in Fig. 2.1a, physical activity has four dimensions including mode/type (walking, running, gardening), frequency, duration and intensity (metabolic demand; light, moderate, vigorous) [19]. Accurate monitoring of activity dimensions is critical for translating epidemiological assessments into prevention strategies. If a health target such as sustained weight loss is associated with moderate-vigorous intensity activity, increasing participation in more intensive activities is suggested. However, if the association is closer with the total physical activity, the public health action would be to encourage physical activity in general. Hence, monitoring the dimension of activity facilitates the design of interventions.

Despite the well-established health benefits of physical activity and the broader national and global impact, many individuals are insufficiently physically active. The deployment of an mhealth platform to promote physical activity necessitates an understanding of aspects affecting the level of physical activities and its sustained maintenance. Research on behavioural strategies has shown that individualising lifestyle interventions based on motivational needs are the main factor to induce an individual to adopt physical activity [16]. To maintain physical activity, self-monitoring [4] and feedback provision [20] are critical behavioural strategies. These requirements are attainable using the remote monitoring aspect of mhealth where personal activity plans will be developed either based on the index of activity by an automated analysis algorithm or a remote coach where needed.

Remote monitoring of physical activity also enables efficient surveillance. The potential of mhealth for surveillance can be mapped to remote monitoring and cloud computing strategic points. This facilitates data collection on physical activity of the community, storage of heavyweight information and data analytics to derive patterns. These patterns help decision makers understand the outcome of different types of interventions, develop predictive models of intervention schemes and better identify suitable strategies with the best health outcomes. A surveillance study by Rovniak et al. [21] identified two major physical activity patterns of adults in two regions of the US. The first pattern emphasises the importance of peer psychosocial support. The social networking aspect of mhealth improves communication between individuals who receive peer advice on their commitment to physical fitness. A second pattern suggests a lack of awareness to be involved in physical activities, particularly vigorous-intensity activities, and hence interventions for encouraging intense activities is desirable. The solution of mhealth for this pattern is information dissemination. Short Message Services (SMS) empower individuals with information and motivation to adopt healthy lifestyles and spread awareness in communities [22]. A third pattern suggests that physical activities are biased towards leisure and occupational domains and the active occupational group is more prone to sedentary lifestyles when not engaged in work. The implication of mhealth for the institutionalisation of physical activity in four domains can be mapped to incorporating economic, social and cognitive behavioural feedback interventions that are specifically tailored to the need of individuals [23–28]. While such interventions provide encouragement and positive reinforcement for the activity, the probability of cheating behaviour, particularly in youth, should be taken into consideration in the design of the platform [29, 30]. The tailorability concept of interventions is also critical to improving compliance. Long et al. [31] developed an algorithm to evaluate the risk of dropping out of the scheme and tailored interventions accordingly to trigger motivation and improve compliance.

To develop a personalised physical activity scheme, quantification of physical activity is essential. As demonstrated in Fig. 2.1b, practitioners have attempted to derive an index of physical activity using various subjective and objective methods [18, 32]. The index of activity can be obtained using self-report questionnaires or diaries [33, 34]. The metric is simple and easy to interoperate; however, it is subjective and lacks validity and reliability due to individual observation and interpretation [35]. Moreover, it is more accurate for assessing vigorous-intensity physical activity rather than light-moderate ones [36, 37]. An objective metric for physical activity assessment is measuring walking steps using pedometers [32]. Commercially available pedometers estimate the walking/running distance and also the time spent in different intensity levels [18]. Although walking is the most common form of activity in the general population, there is a need for a more generic metric to capture various modes of physical activities [38].

An objective index for physical activity quantification is the physical activity energy expenditure (PAEE), where the rate of PAEE is strongly associated with the intensity of physical activity [18]. PAEE is 15–30% of the total energy expenditure (TEE). Resting energy expenditure (REE) and thermic effect of food (TEF) are respectively 60–75% and 10% of TEE [39]. Hills et al. [39] reviewed individual characteristics that determine REE; however, three factors including age, gender and body size, have a significant impact on REE. Typically, the Harris and Benedict equation [40] is used for REE estimation:

– Male

$$REE = 66 + \left(13.7 \times Weight_{kg}\right) + \left(5 \times Height_{cm}\right) - \left(6.8 \times Age_{yrs}\right) \qquad (2.1)$$

– Female

$$REE = 655 + \left(6.9 \times Weight_{kg}\right) + \left(1.8 \times Height_{cm}\right) - \left(6.9 \times Age_{yrs}\right) \qquad (2.2)$$

Consequently, TEF is calculated as:

$$TEF = 0.1 \times REE. \qquad (2.3)$$

Gold standard methods for measuring PAEE are indirect calorimetry [41, 42] and Doubly Labelled Water (DLW) [43, 44] that measure TEE from oxygen consumption and carbon dioxide production followed by deriving PAEE from a formula as explained in Ainslie et al. [45]. The cost and time associated with these laboratory-based methods and the provision of skilled operators are prominent barriers to deployment as mhealth monitoring methods. To address these challenges, portable indirect calorimetry devices have been developed. Although the performance of both Meta-max™ and Cosmed K_4b^2™ have been validated, they have limited use in free-living settings due to their cumbersome and costly nature [45, 46].

In an alternative method, the PAEE can be estimated indirectly using sensors embedded in smartphones or wearables. Because there are many wearable choices available and there is no gold standard, systematic decision-making processing is proposed [18, 32]. The selection methods consider four characteristics of physical activity assessment including study characteristics (budget, population, objectives), population characteristics (age, health status, socio-economic status), instrument characteristics (mode of administration, measured constructs, psychometric properties) and physical activity domain and dimensions. However, exploiting mhealth solutions for physical activity assessment requires a generic platform that integrates the entire characteristics mentioned above. Commonly available sensor technologies rely on either physiological or inertial metrics to derive PAEE.

Estimation of PAEE using physiological metrics is convenient and inexpensive. The main metric of interest is heart rate because it is linearly correlated to oxygen consumption and hence PAEE [47]. With the development of on-body heart rate monitoring sensors, this method of PAEE measurement sounds practical. However, the applicability of this method is mainly limited to moderate-vigorous physical activities [18, 48]. Furthermore, heart rate can be affected by factors besides physical activity and hence requires individual calibration [49]. Another indirect method of measuring PAEE is using motion sensors by converting counts of inertial sensors to energy expenditure units [18, 45]. Physical activity assessment using inertial sensors available in smartphones and on-body sensors is discussed in the next section, as is the challenging endeavour to address the needs of inertial sensors as an optimal physical activity assessment approach.

2.2 Sensor Technologies

For remote monitoring of physical activity, two motion sensor platforms can be incorporated into the lifestyle of individuals. One is inertial sensors embedded in smartphones, wearable sensors and intelligent clothes, and the other is ambient sensors such as infrared (IR) cameras [50, 51]. Although the ambient method provides a remote, passive mode of monitoring, efforts for the deployment in infrastructure such as buildings and or baby cribs is required for the full body monitoring and therefore are beyond the scope of this book.

Monitoring physical activity using inertial sensors (accelerometer and gyroscope) and magnetometers is widely accepted (Fig. 2.2a). Triaxial accelerometers (Triax) are sensitive to acceleration in periodic (vibration), instantaneous (shock) and static (tilt and rotation) modes [52], gyroscopes respond to Coriolis forces and determine the angular velocity and changes in orientation and magnetometers detect the absolute orientation by sensing the strength of the earth's magnetic field [53]. Accelerometers are used typically in conjunction with gyroscopes and/or magnetometers to provide low-cost, quantitative three-dimensional (3D) measurements of body movements.

Recent advances in sensor technologies allow for raw data acquisition at a relatively high sampling frequency (40–100 Hz) that can be processed using native or cloud-based apps to extract the information of interest [32]. Although a low sampling rate is of interest for energy saving, it is prone to excluding signal details. A recent study by Khan et al. [54] suggested an automated method for optimising sampling rates for a specific mode of activity to balance performance and power consumption. Another energy-efficient approach in which the activity is first classified as dynamic or static and then the sampling frequency and window size of classification duration are adapted. This method achieved more than 64% average energy saving and 92% average accuracy in recognising 6 activities [55].

The raw inertial data obtained at an optimised sampling rate is typically expressed in the *counts* per defined time interval (epoch) and the intensity of activity is projected to counts per epoch. The count value is strongly dependent on technical specifications of individual sensors such as A/D conversion scale and frequency filtering range [56]. To standardise the readings of inertial sensors, the sensors are calibrated to convert counts to physiologically meaningful PAEE units including kilocalories or metabolic equivalent (MET) [18, 39] using prediction equations [57–61]. Prediction equations can be obtained from the laboratory-based calibration process against DLW or calorimeters [62].

Since most physical activity recommendations, for example, the 2008 physical activity guidelines for Americans [63], stress the duration and intensity of the physical activity, the PAEE value can be expressed in an alternative metric. For this purpose, thresholds are applied to translate the PAEE value into an intensity-based construct including sedentary (MET: 1–1.5), light (MET: 1.6–2.9), moderate (MET: 3.0–5.9) and vigorous (MET > 6.0) activities [59] (Fig. 2.2b).

To evaluate the validity of the prediction equation, an estimation of inertial sensors of PAEE was compared with the DLW technique over a broad range of datasets [64];

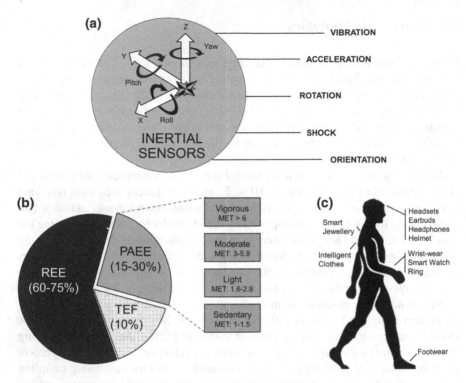

Fig. 2.2 **a** Inertial sensors and detectable motion types, **b** components of total energy expenditure (TEE): Resting energy expenditure (REF), thermic effect of food (TEF) and physical activity energy expenditure (PAEE). PAEE is used as a metric to classify the physical activity based on the intensity into four categories of vigorous, moderate, light and sedentary activity in accordance with the MET (metabolic equivalent) value, **c** the wearability map of inertial sensors

most inertial sensors performed poorly compared to the gold standard of DLW. One factor affecting the accuracy of PAEE estimation using inertial sensors is the limited datasets. To address this issue, Freedson et al. [61] have provided best practice recommendations for researchers. Development of a public access inertial data repository including a broad range of human characteristics (age, gender, body mass and cardiorespiratory fitness) and activities (sedentary lifestyle, sport and leisure activities) is recommended. This provides researchers access to large inertial databases for developing prediction equations.

A second factor affecting the validation studies against DLW is the error associated with prediction equations. In the light of concerns about validation of prediction equations across the continuum of activity dimensions, the development of a single equation across the continuum of population and activities is still a matter of debate. This is due to the inherent limitations of single prediction equations imposed by the calibration approach [65]. A comprehensive study on the performance of commonly used prediction equations by Lyden et al. [56] has identified challenges in the validation of these methods. Prediction equations tend to perform accurately within a specific range of physical activity mode that is used to develop the equation and over/underestimate the energy cost of other activities.

To overcome the limitation of single prediction equations, one recommends a combination with physiological sensors such as heart rate monitors [66]. However, the application of multi-sensor platforms in free-living settings can be limited by factors such as the cost, potential discomfort of wearing multiple sensors for long periods of time and computationally resource-intensive requirements of multisensory platforms [32]. Additionally, developments in the field of inertial sensors is promising. Consequently, there is an emphasis on exploring methods to improve the performance of inertial sensors through the utility of separate estimation equations for different modes of activities.

A two-equation system showed comparable PAEE values relative to DLW [67] and calorimetry [68] in adults. However, a study on youth has shown the performance of single- and two-equation models were not truly equivalent to the calorimetry, although the two-equation system performed relatively more accurately [69]. Besides activity-specific equations, more detailed divisions might be advantageous. Strath et al. [70] evaluated the accuracy and precision of a single prediction equation in three target populations: Children, senior adults and adults with limited functionality. Despite a good agreement across different populations, individual-specific characteristics may enhance the performance of prediction equations. However, it is not known, where appropriate, what population characteristics should be considered as classifying variables. Another study evaluated the importance of disease-specific prediction equations in children with chronic conditions [71].

There are challenges for the development of a multi-equation platform that should be addressed. To switch effectively between equations that each maps to a mode of activity, the count value should meet a threshold condition. However, the count value is integrated over time and does not reflect the profile of activity, and consequently, two activities with a similar integrated count value but different profiles (walking and lifting boxes) results in similar estimates of PAEE [56]. To address this issue, it is proposed to use further features of inertial sensors, such as signal distributions and frequency spectra. Staudenmayer et al. [72] initiated the use of artificial neural networks to identify the mode of activity based on the pattern of inertial sensor signal over time. Further development and refinements have been carried out using other machine learning techniques such as support vector machines [73, 74], hidden Markov models [75] and other types of artificial neural networks [72, 76].

There is extensive research on physical activity recognition where the classifiers are aimed at differentiating various combinations of dynamic and static activities. Physical activity recognition using multiple inertial sensors placed on different parts of the human body results in high performance in terms of accuracy and sensitivity [77–79]. However, a multi-sensor platform may reduce compliance due to obstructiveness; hence, a single sensor monitoring system is desirable. Mathie et al. [80] suggested a 2-stage classification using a single triaxial accelerometer in which activities are first labelled as activity and rest, followed by a classification of the activity category. The work was followed by Ravi et al. [81] by increasing the variety of activities and assessing the potential of a single inertial sensor. In more recent years, emerging advanced sensor technologies have shifted towards smartphones and wearables. Kwapisz et al. [82] evaluated the performance of a smartphone-based accelerometer to recognise six physical activities. Woznowski et al. [83] systematically reviewed existing sensor technologies for activity recognition to understand technological requirements for a specific activity. Current methods of activity recognition have evolved to the point that they can be considered ready for being part of routine clinical monitoring. Additionally, anti-cheating algorithms have been developed [30]. Nonetheless, there are challenges for the development of this paradigm as an assistive clinical tool.

Conventional methods of activity recognition are based on static features that limit the generalisability of the system across users and activity modes [84]. Deep learning has the potential to leverage a dynamic approach for adaptive activity learning and improve the performance for new users of a system or to identify new behaviour of a known user [85]. Hammerla et al. [86] assessed the performance of three methods including deep feed-forward networks, conventional networks and recurrent networks; the latter two experienced less variability across data sets. Recurrent networks (Long Short-Term Memory cells [87]) outperformed other methods by a significant margin particularly in long-term, repetitive activities by exploiting the temporal dependencies. A more recent study by Le et al. [88] reported the use of a Sequential Forward Feature Selection algorithm to recognise 19 daily activities with the average classification accuracy of 99.91%. Although significant progress in the field of activity mode recognition has been made, there are challenges for the advancement of the field that should be addressed. These challenges include improving the performance in naturalistic environments and enhancing the sensitivity of activity recognition methods across the entire spectrum of activity types, including low-speed walking.

Although the activity classification methods appear to be successful in laboratory-based settings, their validity decreases in a free-living environment. This implies that independent datasets from real-world settings are required to develop and validate the classifiers to assure they are transportable to other datasets. Previous studies have shown the improvement in performance of activity recognition methods using free-living datasets [89, 90]. An alternative method is a semi population-based approach in which activity models are developed using a training dataset and models are adapted to a new user using a small dataset [91].

The sensitivity of activity classifiers is considerably limited in a range of physical activities, such as low-speed walking and non-ambulatory activities, such as cycling, weight lifting and steps [32, 92, 93]. The performance of inertial sensors at low-speed walking is deficient; the gait speed in seniors with frailty syndrome and a mean age of above 82 is less than 0.75 m/s [94, 95]. Previous studies on step detection using a single sensor for this target group resulted in a minimum 19.1% error [96–98]. Increasing the number of sensors or wearing a single sensor on the ankle can enhance the performance at the cost of decreasing compliance due to discomfort [99–101]. A recent study improved the performance of step detection algorithms in low-speed walking using a single waist-wear sensor and achieved an error of 10%, with a mean sensitivity of 99% [102]. Although the validity of the proposed algorithm for other wearing modes was not evaluated, the outcome sounds promising.

Elevating the performance of inertial sensors to detect and monitor non-ambulatory activities is an ongoing research theme. Of those static activities, cycling has attracted attention as a popular mode of short-distance transportation and a recreational activity [103]. However, the variations in population and activity intensity result in a relatively low classification rate [104]. With a focus on activity recognition independent of intensity, Alshurafa et al. [105] proposed a robust method which included stochastic activity modelling and stochastic approximation decision. Bonomi et al. [106] have shown that appropriate feature engineering has the potential to elevate the performance. The uncertainties involved in the classification can be addressed by a Fuzzy Logic approach; Fahimi et al. [107] showed a significant improvement in the accuracy of static activity recognition.

The aforementioned studies have shown that for limited known sensor placements, inertial sensors have the capability to classify physical activities [108]. This implies that activity recognition methods rely on the knowledge of sensor placement, which is not a priori in practical applications [109]. The functionality of inertial sensors for body movement studies depends critically on the placement and orientation of the sensor; even a slight displacement of the sensor from its reference position might decrease the accuracy of signal acquisition. Imposing placement constraints could reduce the complexity. The *wearability map* (Fig. 2.2c) suggests an ergonomic guideline for sensor placement on a human body including collar area, forearm, waist and top of the foot [110]. However, the strategy of sensor placement constraints is not applicable for two main reasons: First, inertial sensors are available in a wide range of devices with various modes of wearability and second, such a strategy challenges practical compliance.

Inertial sensors are currently available in different modes, including embedded in smartphones and wearables or woven into intelligent clothes [111]. The smartphone plays the role of an interface for the on-body sensors (wearable and textile). Wearable sensors can be directly attached to the body in the form of self-sticker [112, 113] or by straps [114], wristbands (Fitbit® [115], Microsoft-band™ [116], UP2® [117], Nike FuelBand® [118]) or other accessories such as headsets/earbuds/headphones [119, 120], helmet [121] and shoes [122]. There are detailed reviews on wearable sensors which compare their algorithms, communication protocols, materials and safety; however, the issues relating to the user-acceptability and compliance are neglected [123–125]. Although the wearing time of wearables depends on the lifestyle and the type of physical activity, a study on the comfort of wearable sensors has been carried out.

A 24/7 study of physical activity monitoring of women aged 30–64 using hip-, upper arm- and wrist-wear sensors showed that the wrist-wear with ~95% wearing time was the most acceptable mode, followed by upper arm-wear and hip-wear [126]. The outcome of this study confirmed another pilot study comparing hip- and wrist-wear accelerometers, where the wrist-wear one achieved a higher compliance [127]. Besides comfort, these findings are in line with the aesthetics taste of users as well as concerns about ambient overload [128]. Emphasis on suppressing the impact of screen and object awareness leads the design of wearable sensors towards intelligent jewelleries [129], such as a smart ring (Oura [130]). An alternative to smart jewellery is intelligent clothes. Advances in sensor development and material science have resulted in miniaturised, low-cost, low-energy and more accurate inertial sensors that can be integrated into garments [124]. Examples of intelligent clothes for physical activity assessment are available in the literature including BIOSWIM® [131], WEALTHY® [132], MagIC® [133], a prototype developed by Naizmand et al. [134], MERMOTH® [135], VTAMN® [136] and MyHeart® [137]. Although this mode of monitoring enables incorporating more than one inertial sensor node and therefore the accuracy of measurements improves [138], its cumbersome feature limits compliance in long-term monitoring.

Constraining the placement of on-body sensors limits flexibility and hence does not chime with the mhealth attributes of convenience, user-acceptability and compliance. The optimal body location for the inertial sensor is still a subject of debate [139, 140]. However, most studies have recommended waist-wear because it is close to the centre of the human body (the torso) and thereby more accurate signals are acquired for assessing whole-body movements [62, 140, 141]. However, waist-wear instruments are not desirable in terms of convenience and obstructiveness. Previous studies on compliance based on the percentage of wear time have shown 25% compliance for a waist-wear accelerometer versus above 70% for a wrist-wear accelerometer [141]. Wrist-wear instruments, however, might be prone to systematic errors due to random hand movements. Gjoreski et al. [142] evaluated the performance of a wrist-wear device for activity recognition. They showed that the performance of the non-dominant hand can outperform that of other locations via feature engineering. In the case of driving data stream from embedded inertial sensors into smartphones, investigating the optimum placement of the smartphone has shown the difference in accuracy between locations [143]. However, the results are reasonably close to practical applications and optimising the methodology by feature engineering may further improve the accuracy [144, 145].

In a parallel attempt to feature engineering, automatic localisation techniques are considered to recognise the placement of inertial sensors on the human body. These techniques consist of two stages; in the first stage, the walking segments are automatically detected, and algorithms in the second stage use the walking patterns to detect the position of the sensor [146–149]. The existing localisation methods have achieved an accuracy of above 90% in the placement recognition of the inertial sensors in accordance with the wearability map. Likewise, the localisation methods are developed for locating the position of a smartphone on the body, in case embedded inertial sensors are used; for a further discussion see the review by del Rosario et al. [150]. Though the majority of these studies were focused on the localisation of accelerometers, methods for the calibration of magnetometers have also been proposed [151–154]. It should be noted that the method of sensor localisation necessitates a pre-processing step which might be computationally expensive to execute on a smartphone and hence a cloud-based approach is recommended.

Given the promising results of feature engineering and sensor localisation, a combined method might lead to a robust dynamic data acquisition approach. This neces-

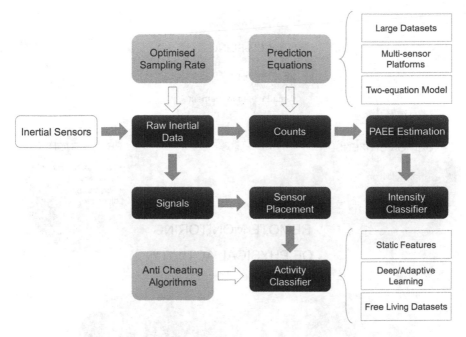

Fig. 2.3 Flowchart for remote monitoring of physical activity using mhealth solutions

sitates conducting further pilot studies to optimise the process of feature extraction, in both time and frequency domains, by incorporating free-living training databases. These features are then extracted from the acquired data streams of inertial sensors in the test phase and processed to detect the sensor placement and optimise data validity. Figure 2.3 illustrates a generic algorithm for remote monitoring of physical activity including PAEE estimator and activity classifier.

2.3 Clinical Value

The notion of "physical activity as medicine" projects the substantial benefits of regular physical activity in well-being, longevity and sustainable healthcare systems [155] (Fig. 2.4). The impact of implementation of mhealth interventions on enhancing and maintaining physical activity has been well established in limited and global pilot studies [20, 156–159]. As discussed in previous sections, the key enabling technologies for the deployment of such an mhealth platform are high-performance miniaturised inertial sensors and intelligent biosignal processing algorithms that ultimately underpin adapting physically active lifestyles.

A promising approach for promoting physical activity is integrating remote activity monitoring with the game industry to develop interactive video games, namely

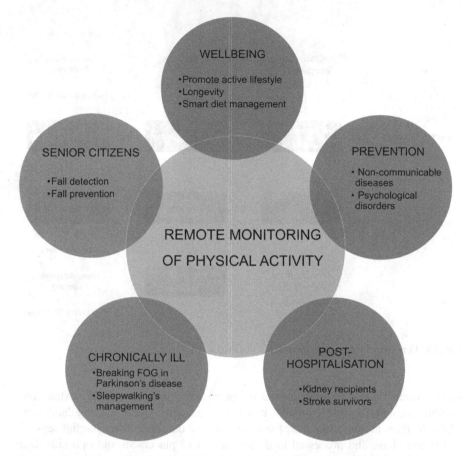

Fig. 2.4 The quintant of remote physical activity monitoring across the wellbeing continuum

exergames [160]. Evidence for the efficacy of exergames are driven from clinical trials carried out in youths and adults. Baranowski et al. [161] studied what enhancing physical activity does in children aged 10–12 years. Furthermore, clinical trials evaluated the impact of interactive games on the health status of senior citizens and showed significant progress in physical and cognitive skills [162–167]. The underlying cause of adherence to structured activity plans delivered through exergames is that the individual is rewarded in the game and can achieve tangible virtual outcomes; therefore, the activity per se is not the focus of attention [168]. To enhance the compliance further, this experience can become more enjoyable by using virtual reality headsets such as Oculus Rift™ that create an illusion of presence [169].

This section provides an overview of the benefits of institutionalizing physical activity through mhealth interventions using smartphones and wearable sensors for remote physical monitoring.

2.3.1 Dietary Management

Remote monitoring of physical activity enables the measurements of energy expenditure in daily living conditions which can be widely adopted as a criterion method for dietary management. Poor dietary habits are correlated with an increased prevalence of obesity [170–172] and long-term health conditions such as DM and cancer [173–178]. Intelligent technologies, including image-based apps [179], smart fork [180], smart tray [181] and smart tablecloths [182], have been developed to identify eating habits (eating speed, bite volume and patterns) and nutrition intake. However, the value of these methods is limited unless the energy expenditure of the individual is taken into account to provide personalised dietary recommendations. The emerging Internet-of-Things provides a smart infrastructure that connects food assessment sensors to remote activity monitoring solutions. In the future, integrating smart fridges [183–185], smart packages [186], e-commerce and automated grocery shops [187] into this platform should allow a tailored food menu planning based on the health needs of an individual and developing the "Internet of Food" [188]. Such an intelligent system could also incorporate the health condition of the individual into the decision making process to check for specific entities; for example, peanuts for food allergies, carbohydrate consumption for DM or saturated fats for CVD [188].

2.3.2 Premature Mortality

Arem et al. [189] evaluated the impact of leisure-time physical activity dose on premature mortality rate where the dose is the total volume of energy consumption per unit time. According to the 2008 Physical Activity Guidelines for Americans [63], a minimum of 7.5 MET hours per week is required for substantial health benefits. Adherence to the minimum recommended physical activity leads to a 31% decrease in premature mortality. The premature mortality risk is minimised at 39% for approximately 3–5 times the recommended physical activity (22.5–40 MET).

2.3.3 Non-communicable Diseases

Physical activity is one of the top four evidence-based global targets to reduce non-communicable diseases [190]. The decrease in the index of physical activity in individuals with COPD results in a higher risk of hospitalisation and premature death. To avoid these risks, the feasibility of enhancing and maintaining physical activity using mhealth interventions in COPD patients was evaluated [191]. The outcome of this pilot study showed that the proposed intervention has a positive impact on stimulating behavioural drivers and eventually the index of physical activity, health status and life quality of participants.

In line with a global trend to shift from CVD treatment to prevention, physical activity is highly endorsed as a prevention policy [192, 193]. CVD accounts for 17.3M deaths per year and this is expected to increase to more than 23.6 M by 2030 [190]. Accordingly, the American Heart Association has considered promoting a physically active lifestyle as 1 of the 7 goals for cardiovascular health in 2020 [194]. A review by Kokkinos [195] provides an insight into the correlation between dimensions of physical activity and premature mortality rate due to CVD. Accordingly, the intensity of activity plays a more critical role in the risk reduction than the duration of activity. However, the interaction between dimensions of physical activity provides the flexibility in the design of structured programs of physical activity across age groups and health conditions. A noteworthy finding is that physical activity potentially provides a greater degree of cardiovascular health benefits for women than men, resulting in a 38% lower cardiovascular mortality rate [196, 197].

Evidence from several studies confirms the impact of physical activity on reducing the mortality risk in individuals with hypertension [198–200]. Performing physical activity of >5 MET reduces the risk of premature mortality between 34 and 70%. Faselis et al. [201] examined the association between physical activity and mortality rate across the BMI continuum; each 1 MET increase in physical activity results in 20, 12 and 25% mortality risk reduction for respectively BMI < 25 (normal), 25 < BMI < 29.9 (overweight) and BMI > 35 (obese).

The currently available pilot studies and clinical trials have shown that a significant impact of physical activity on delaying or averting the development of Type 2 DM (T2DM) [202–210]. A prevention study achieved a 58% risk reduction in T2DM by promoting physical activity [211], where self-monitoring plays a critical role [212]. Tailoring mhealth interventions to promote physical activity in individuals with T2DM necessitates understanding their risk perception and allowing for emotions, cognition and behaviour [213]. A systematic study by Wareham et al. [214] with an aim of developing a prevention strategy showed the strong relationship between physical activity and insulin resistance. However, quantification of benefits is subject to future studies. A meta-analysis by Aune et al. [215] identified the association between dimensions of physical activity and the relative risks (RR) of high versus low activity. The summary of RR values incorporating various physical activity intensities (vigorous, moderate and low) and total physical activity, respectively, were between 0.61 and 0.68. Another noteworthy finding was the observed non-linear relationship between the physical activity dose and T2DM with an exponential decay, implying a more noticeable decay at low dose values. The importance of physical activity on DM risks is observed equally across race/ethnic groups [216]; however, racial epidemiological findings demonstrate activity-related reduction of T2DM is more pronounced in Caucasians than Afro-Caribbeans [195]. A systematic review by Sigal et al. identified that performing both aerobic and resistance activities is the optimal mode of activity with a minimum duration of 150 min/week [217]. Waden et al. [218] explored the potential of leisure-time physical activity to suppress late complications of Type 1 DM (T1DM), particularly nephropathy. A meta-analysis of the protective effect of physical activity on gestational DM (prevalence of 2–10% in the US) identified an average of 28% risk reduction [219].

2.3.4 Psychological Disorders

Integrating physical activity in daily lives through mhealth solutions also provides sufficient capacity to curb the burden of psychological disorders. A study on the burden of disease in 2030 identified depressive disorder as one of the leading causes of DALYs worldwide [220]. Encouraging physical activity can reduce depression in adolescents and adults by enhancing self-esteem and social support [221–224]. Evidence suggests the association with total physical activity is more pronounced than that with the intensity of activity [221]. Besides unipolar depression, the impact of physical activity on a spectrum of psychological and somatoform disorders is evident [225–228]. The indirect benefits of physical activity in patients with cognitive impairment such as dementia are related to slowing down the deterioration of functional performance, particularly reducing the fall risk [229–231]. The prevalence of dementia in 2015 was estimated at ~47M and it is projected to double every 20 years and reach 131.5M in 2050 [232]. Accordingly, it is essential to deploy remote solutions for encouraging structured physical activity that provides a lifestyle intervention enabling individuals to maintain a high quality of life in the community. A meta-analysis of physical activity on autism spectrum disorder (ASD) determined the constructive impact of individual activity interventions on enhancing social integration and motor skills [233]. Besides therapeutic potential, individual activity interventions can be considered as a prevention paradigm in ASD. Remote activity monitoring of youths with ASD using inertial sensors indicated that sedentary behaviour is more prevalent in adolescents than children [234]. Therefore, stimulating and maintaining general activity from an early age can avert health, academic and social consequences in adolescent years [235].

2.3.5 Post-discharge Management

Clinical benefits of the implementation of smart activity monitoring platforms are beyond wellness and prevention categories of the patient pathway. Remote monitoring of physical activity can also benefit newly discharged patients. Clinical trials by Lorenz et al. [236] have shown that stimulating physical activity after kidney transplantation holds potential promise to improve the survival rate of recipients. In their study, adherence to the recommended physical activity was ~36% which could be caused by using a pedometer instead of a smart sensor (smartphone/on-body sensor) and lack of personalised lifestyle interventions by text messages over the period of study. Clinical trials are required to evaluate boosting adherence and following the socioeconomic effectiveness of using multiple aspects of mhealth. Physical activity monitoring with an emphasis on arm movements is beneficial to stroke survivors. Leuenberger et al. [237] developed a wrist-ware sensor to monitor affected-arm movements and facilitate retention of arm function through tailoring the rehabilitation scheme.

2.3.6   Fall Detection and Fall Prevention

Remote monitoring of physical activity provides management solutions for at risk senior adults particularly those living alone or in remote areas, and also adults with long-term health conditions, such as multiple sclerosis. A smart motion sensor platform with a fall detection feature is beneficial to senior adults who live alone in the community. According to epidemiological studies in the UK [238], about 33% of individuals aged over 75 experience a fall each year and globally one in three people over age 65 have one fall or more each year [239–242]. Hospital admissions for fall-related injuries in people over age 65 varies between 10 and 40% [242–244], depending on how fall-related injuries are defined [245]. The burden of fall-related injuries is projected to rise significantly by 2060 given the global demographic trends; for example, 24.2% of people in the UK will be over 65 by 2040 [246], 25% of the population in the US will be over age 85 by 2030 [247] and in Europe, 40 and 11% will be over age 65 and 80, respectively [191]. Moreover, solo living is rising; in the UK the number of people living alone increased by ~10% between 2001 and 2011 [248].

The associated fall-related consequences are significant; for example, hip fracture leads to an average hospitalisation-days of 5.9 [249], a four-fold increase in nursing-need and more than two-fold increase in premature mortality [250]. Although the majority of falls do not cause injury, they might pose severe risks to the quality of life, such as restricting daily and social activities due to fear of falling [251, 252]. Fall-related injuries also place the economic burden on society. The management of injurious falls in 2000 is estimated to cost US$19B [253] and AU$2.3B [254] in the US and Australia, respectively.

Remote motion monitoring can address the healthcare burden of fall-related injuries through two approaches: Fall detection and fall prevention. The fall detection solution triggers rapid assistance, i.e. alerting emergency services following a fall to improve the patient's outcome, particularly in the case of solo living; ~50% of senior adults are not able to get up after fall [255]. The main contributor to fall-related injuries is the time the person remains on the ground following a fall. In 20% of falls, this time, exceeds one hour [256], resulting in associated complications such as dehydration, hypothermia, bronchopneumonia and pressure sores [255, 257]. Moreover, the lag time above an hour in severe falls is correlated to 50% rate of premature mortality within six months [256].

Fall detectors were initially introduced as wrist-worn accelerometers [258] and later in line with the implementation of mhealth, smartphone-based fall detectors have been developed and continue to make more advanced progress [259–264]. Unsupervised fall detection algorithms process the acquired data from inertial sensors to detect falls based on *fall features*. Previous researches on supervised feature extraction and feature reduction suggests a set of discriminative features to classify fall and non-fall (daily) activities while the probabilities of false positive and false negatives are minimised. The performance of existing fall detection solutions including fall features (magnitude, mean and standard deviation of acceleration [260, 265],

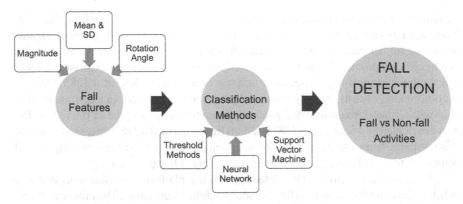

Fig. 2.5 Remote monitoring of fall detection using the mhealth platform

rotation angle [265, 266]) and classification methods (threshold method [260, 265], neural networks [267–269] and support vector machine [266, 270]) are reviewed extensively [262, 271, 272] (Fig. 2.5). Developing an ideal set of fall features is still an ongoing research objective, whereas a recent study has shown the superiority of support vector machines [273].

Although existing algorithms can exhibit both sensitivity and specificity of 100% in experimental setups, their performance deteriorates in real-world settings [271]. Bagalà et al. [274] assessed the performance of 13 existing fall detection algorithms in real-world settings; the average sensitivity and specificity of high-performance algorithms can plunge between 57 and 83%, respectively. Moreover, the number of false alarms was too many to be acceptable in the real-world [274]. To address these issues, two approaches have been suggested: The development of a real-world fall database to improve the performance of existing algorithms and developing adaptive algorithms [274–276]. The improved fall detection platform promises benefits to vulnerable senior adults by timely detection of fall and ultimately reduces the related healthcare costs and mortality rate [277].

The fall prevention solution predicts an increased risk of fall by detecting a deterioration in functional ability based on a set of controlled physical activities including a Sit-to-Stand test, an Alternate Step Test and a Time-Up-and-Go test [278–281]. These tests can be performed in unsupervised, real-world settings. In a pilot study, Mathie et al. [282] assessed the feasibility of long-term remote activity monitoring where adults aged between 80 and 86 carried out the test every day for 2–3 months. The instructions were paper-based; however, mhealth allows the development of an interactive app for a visual/audio guideline. This app also enables setting reminders while, at the same time, it empowers healthcare provider to make amendments based on the cloud-based health record and communicates with the user at the third place.

Podsiadlo et al. [281] used the Time-Up-and-Go test wherein the timed measure determines the risk of fall; Shumway-Cook et al. [283] suggested a cut-off point of 13.5 s for predicting fall risk. However, this timing measure is not sufficiently sensitive for clinical purposes. Zakaria et al. [284] divided the test into phases of basic activity such as walking, turning and sitting and processed the acquired signals to extract further parameters to evaluate fall risk while providing extra knowledge for the healthcare provider with the analysis of the performance in each phase. Another comprehensive semi-supervised approach was proposed by Menz et al. [285] wherein a combination of tests, namely directed-routine, are performed. In a continuation of this work, time-domain directed-routine parameters that can predict the risk of fall were extracted and optimised [278] and then Redmond et al. [286] processed acquired data streams from inertial sensors by segmentation to convert the semi-supervised approach to a trustworthy and reliable unsupervised fall risk analyser.

The adoption of remote fall-related monitoring platforms enables independence while enhancing the sense of safety for senior adults living alone. The outcome of surveys have shown that the technology is acceptable among this age group [287–290]; however, there are adoption barriers such as privacy [291] and social stigmatisation [287]. From a privacy viewpoint, while a better understanding of the technology reduces concerns, on-body sensors are more desirable than ambient ones such as IR cameras [288, 291]. In terms of stigmatisation, on-body sensors are becoming ubiquitous and now have broad appeal across all age groups; this facilitates the design of an adoption structure among senior adults. Nonetheless, it is essential to integrate ethical and social considerations of senior adults within the engineering cycle to enhance technology acceptance [292, 293]. Moreover, a scoping review strongly encourages the involvement of senior adults in the development chain of fall detection and preventions systems to enhance outcomes [294]. As the feasibility study by Sprute et al. [295] has shown, integrating a fall prevention/detection system into a building can develop a smart, safe environment for senior citizens, particularly those living alone and in remote areas.

Another population of adults that could benefit from the fall prevention platform are individuals with multiple sclerosis (fall prevalence >52%) [296], people with dementia [297, 298] and cancer patients aged over 65 [299] which may experience a higher risk of fall [300]. Apart from vulnerable senior citizens and at-risk patients, the fall prevention platform can be modified to assess driving skills of senior adults [301]; a cut-off point of 9 s in the Rapid Pace Walk [302] test can discriminate high-risk senior drivers [301].

2.3.7 Sleepwalking

The remote motion monitoring platform has the capability to support sleepwalking patients in a smart house. Although sleepwalking (somnambulism) is more common in children, its prevalence in adults is ~2–15% [303, 304]. Episodes of sleepwalking that last between 30 s and 30 min [305] may lead to unpredictable safety incidents, social embarrassment and anxiety [305]. Singhal and Jain [306] developed an accelerometer-based monitoring system to execute an alarm code whenever an event is detected. The alarm aims to regain patient's conscious and also alert first-to-contact by a call on one registered mobile number together with a message including the location based on the GPS data. This area of remote movement monitoring is less established compared to others and thus further pilot studies are required to explore applicable aspects of mhealth.

2.3.8 Parkinson's Disease

Individuals with Parkinson's disease (PD) also can drive benefit from the implementation of the smart movement sensor platform. PD, following Alzheimer's disease, is the second most common neurodegenerative disorder worldwide [307] and its prevalence rises with age; between 0.1 and 1.9% for individuals 50–59 and over 80, respectively [308]. A study on the burden of PD in the US in 2010 has shown that 630,000 PD patients imposed a direct cost of US$14B and an indirect cost of U$6.3B [309]. According to demographic studies this burden is expected to double by 2040 in the US [309]. Remote movement monitoring can also be applied as a diagnostic support tool to detect PD symptoms [310], a remote monitoring approach to observe changes in PD symptoms in response to therapy [311] or a management strategy to detect freeze of gait and adopt effective unfreezing interventions.

One of the common symptoms of Parkinson's disease is a freeze of gait (FOG) with a prevalence of ~40% after 10 years [312]. FOG is a gait disorder characterised by a "sudden and transient" [313] difficulty in walking as if the feet "were glued to the floor" [314] which increases the risk of falls [315] because of postural instability [316]. PD patients experience FOG mainly in narrow spaces like walking through doorways, turning and encountering obstacles [317]. Because of its unpredictable and variable nature, FOG is correlated with poor life quality and profound loss of independence and mobility [318]. The main clinical benefit of remote movement monitoring is the real-time detection of the onset of the FOG episodes [319]. Breaking the cycle of freezing by visual or rhythmic auditory cues enables the person to walk quite normally and ultimately elevate their life quality with enabling functional independence [320–323].

The performance of a system consisting of a wearable accelerometer for automatic detection of FOG and a wireless headset for stimulating auditory cues to break FOG showed the feasibility of this approach [324]. In line with mhealth characteristics, the customised sensor platform is replaced by a smartphone in more recent studies [325–327]. To improve the performance of real-time FOG detection, previous studies assessed the enhancement in sensitivity, specificity and accuracy of detecting FOG by incorporating advanced signal processing [328], machine learning [325] methods, wavelet transform [329] and Fuzzy Logic [330]. Still, the performance of existing FOG detection methods can be improved to achieve a higher accuracy and instantaneous unfreezing triggers. Moreover, personalised FOG breaking strategies, such as those based on step frequency may boost the effectiveness [331].

In the light of implementation in unsupervised environments, Mazilu et al. [332] carried out a pilot study to investigate the acceptability and impact of an automatic, closed-loop FOG detector with an auditory FOG breaking strategy. The outcome of this study showed that exploiting FOG detection and unfreezing strategies can be successfully employed to alleviate the burden of FOG and eventually improve the life quality of PD individuals. This finding will be further supported by the use of algorithms with enhanced performance and a wider range of real-world experiments by increasing the number of participants and environments with various obstacles [333]. In this context, research on improving the outcome of the PD assistance platform is on-going; sensitivity and specificity of above 90% are achieved [331, 334].

2.3.9 Sports Science

The application of remote activity monitoring can be extended to the realm of sports engineering to offer new insights to enhance the performance and experience of players. The advantage of implementing wrist-wear inertial sensors for monitoring team performance of basketball players was evaluated by Bai et al. [335]. The proposed platform achieved a high accuracy in detecting shoots and the shooter. Wearable inertial sensors for remote activity monitoring are also beneficial to athletes and explorers in challenging environmental conditions such as mountain climbers in Mount Everest [336].

References

1. Williams PT (2004) Vigorous exercise and the population distribution of body weight. Int J Obes 28(1):120–128
2. Weinsier RL, Hunter GR, Desmond RA, Byrne NM, Zuckerman PA, Darnell BE (2002) Free-living activity energy expenditure in women successful and unsuccessful at maintaining a normal body weight. Am J Clin Nutr 75(3):499–504
3. Hill JO, Wyatt HR (2005) Role of physical activity in preventing and treating obesity. J Appl Physiol 99(2):765–770
4. Forman EM, Butryn ML (2016) Effective weight loss: an acceptance-based behavioral approach, clinician guide. Oxford University Press, UK
5. Pi-Sunyer FX, Becker D, Bouchard C, Carleton R, Colditz G, Dietz W, Foreyt J, Garrison R, Grundy S, Hansen B (1998) Clinical guidelines on the identification, evaluation, and treatment of overweight and obesity in adults. Am J Clin Nutr 68(4):899–917
6. Mensink M, Feskens E, Saris W, De Bruin T, Blaak E (2003) Study on lifestyle intervention and impaired glucose tolerance maastricht (SLIM): preliminary results after one year. Int J Obes 27(3):377–384
7. Schellenberg ES, Dryden DM, Vandermeer B, Ha C, Korownyk C (2013) Lifestyle interventions for patients with and at risk for type 2 diabetes: a systematic review and meta-analysis. Ann Intern Med 159(8):543–551
8. Yoon U, Kwok LL, Magkidis A (2013) Efficacy of lifestyle interventions in reducing diabetes incidence in patients with impaired glucose tolerance: a systematic review of randomized controlled trials. Metabolism 62(2):303–314
9. Berlin JA, Colditz GA (1990) A meta-analysis of physical activity in the prevention of coronary heart disease. Am J Epidemiol 132(4):612–628

10. Blair SN, Kampert JB, Kohl HW, Barlow CE, Macera CA, Paffenbarger RS, Gibbons LW (1996) Influences of cardiorespiratory fitness and other precursors on cardiovascular disease and all-cause mortality in men and women. JAMA 276(3):205–210

11. Eckel RH, Krauss RM, Committee AN (1998) American Heart Association call to action: obesity as a major risk factor for coronary heart disease. Circulation 97(21):2099–2100

12. Bergström A, Pisani P, Tenet V, Wolk A, Adami HO (2001) Overweight as an avoidable cause of cancer in Europe. Int J Cancer 91(3):421–430

13. Department of Health and Human Services of United States (1996) Physical activity and health: a report of the Surgeon General. DIANE Publishing, USA

14. WHO (2014) Global strategy on diet, Physical activity and health. http://www.who.int/dietp hysicalactivity/pa/en/. Accessed Dec 2016

15. Chenoweth D, Leutzinger J (2006) The economic cost of physical inactivity and excess weight in American adults. J Phys Act Health 3(2):148–163

16. Seefeldt V, Malina RM, Clark MA (2002) Factors affecting levels of physical activity in adults. Sports Med 32(3):143–168

17. U.S. Department of Health and Human Services (2008) Physical activity guidelines advisory committee report 2008: A1–H14

18. Strath SJ, Kaminsky LA, Ainsworth BE, Ekelund U, Freedson PS, Gary RA, Richardson CR, Smith DT, Swartz AM (2013) Guide to the assessment of physical activity: clinical and research applications a scientific statement from the American heart association. Circulation 128(20):2259–2279

19. Bouchard C, Katzmarzyk P (2000) Physical activity and obesity, 2nd edn. Human Kinetics, UA

20. Hurling R, Catt M, De Boni M, Fairley B, Hurst T, Murray P, Richardson A, Sodhi J (2007) Using internet and mobile phone technology to deliver an automated physical activity program: randomized controlled trial. J Med Internet Res 9(2):e7

21. Rovniak LS, Sallis JF, Saelens BE, Frank LD, Marshall SJ, Norman GJ, Conway TL, Cain KL, Hovell MF (2010) Adults' physical activity patterns across life domains: cluster analysis with replication. Health Psychol 29(5):496–505

22. Stephens J, Allen J (2013) Mobile phone interventions to increase physical activity and reduce weight: a systematic review. J Cardiovasc Nurs 28(4):320–329

23. Pratt M, Macera CA, Sallis JF, O'Donnell M, Frank LD (2004) Economic interventions to promote physical activity: application of the SLOTH model. Am J Prev Med 27(3):136–145

24. Adams MA, Sallis JF, Norman GJ, Hovell MF, Hekler EB, Perata E (2013) An adaptive physical activity intervention for overweight adults: a randomized controlled trial. PLoS ONE 8(12):e82901

25. Anderson I, Maitland J, Sherwood S, Barkhuus L, Chalmers M, Hall M, Brown B, Muller H (2007) Shakra: tracking and sharing daily activity levels with unaugmented mobile phones. Mobile Netw Appl 12(2–3):185–199

26. Tsai CC, Lee G, Raab F, Norman GJ, Sohn T, Griswold WG, Patrick K (2007) Usability and feasibility of PmEB: a mobile phone application for monitoring real time caloric balance. Mobile Netw Appl 12(2–3):173–184

27. Bort-Roig J, Gilson ND, Puig-Ribera A, Contreras RS, Trost SG (2014) Measuring and influencing physical activity with smartphone technology: a systematic review. Sports Med 44(5):671–686

28. Gilson ND, Burton NW, Van Uffelen JG, Brown WJ (2011) Occupational sitting time: employees? perceptions of health risks and intervention strategies. Health Promot J Austr 22(1):38–43

29. Kirby J, Tibbins C, Callens C, Lang B, Thorogood M, Tigbe W, Robertson W (2012) Young people's views on accelerometer use in physical activity research: findings from a user involvement investigation. ISRN obesity. https://doi.org/10.5402/2012/948504

30. Alshurafa N, Eastwood J-A, Pourhomayoun M, Nyamathi S, Bao L, Mortazavi B, Sarrafzadeh M (2014) Anti-cheating: Detecting self-inflicted and impersonator cheaters for remote health monitoring systems with wearable sensors. In: 11th International conference on wearable and implantable body sensor networks, Zurich, Switzerland, 16–19 Jun 2014

31. Long X, Pijl M, Pauws S, Lacroix J, Goris AH, Aarts RM (2014) Towards tailored physical activity health intervention: predicting dropout participants. Health Technol 4(3):273–287
32. Ainsworth B, Cahalin L, Buman M, Ross R (2015) The current state of physical activity assessment tools. Prog Cardiovasc Dis 57(4):387–395
33. Wareham NJ, Jakes RW, Rennie KL, Schuit J, Mitchell J, Hennings S, Day NE (2003) Validity and repeatability of a simple index derived from the short physical activity questionnaire used in the European Prospective Investigation into Cancer and Nutrition (EPIC) study. Public Health Nutr 6(4):407–413
34. Ainsworth BE, Coleman KJ (2006) Physical activity measurement. Taylor & Francis, USA
35. van Poppel MN, Chinapaw MJ, Mokkink LB, Van Mechelen W, Terwee CB (2010) Physical activity questionnaires for adults. Sports Med 40(7):565–600
36. Strath SJ, Bassett DR, Swartz AM (2004) Comparison of the college alumnus questionnaire physical activity index with objective monitoring. Ann Epidemiol 14(6):409–415
37. Ainsworth BE, Richardson MT, Jacobs DR, Leon AS, Sternfeld B (1999) Accuracy of recall of occupational physical activity by questionnaire. J Clin Epidemiol 52(3):219–227
38. Saris W, Binkhorst R (1977) The use of pedometer and actometer in studying daily physical activity in man. Part I: reliability of pedometer and actometer. Eur J Appl Physiol Occup Physiol 37(3):219–228
39. Hills AP, Mokhtar N, Byrne NM (2014) Assessment of physical activity and energy expenditure: An overview of objective measures. Front Nutr. https://doi.org/10.3389/fnut.2014.0 0005. Accessed Oct 2017
40. Roza AM, Shizgal HM (1984) The Harris Benedict equation reevaluated: resting energy requirements and the body cell mass. Am J Clin Nutr 40(1):168–182
41. Haugen HA, Chan L-N, Li F (2007) Indirect calorimetry: a practical guide for clinicians. Nutr Clin Pract 22(4):377–388
42. da Rocha EEM, Alves VGF, da Fonseca RBV (2006) Indirect calorimetry: methodology, instruments and clinical application. Curr Opin Clin Nutr Metab Care 9(3):247–256
43. Schoeller DA, Ravussin E, Schutz Y, Acheson KJ, Baertschi P, Jequier E (1986) Energy expenditure by doubly labeled water: validation in humans and proposed calculation. Am J Physiol Regul Integr Comp Physiol 250(5):R823–R830
44. Schoeller D, Van Santen E (1982) Measurement of energy expenditure in humans by doubly labeled water method. J Appl Physiol 53(4):955–959
45. Ainslie PN, Reilly T, Westerterp KR (2003) Estimating human energy expenditure. Sports Med 33(9):683–698
46. Macfarlane DJ (2001) Automated metabolic gas analysis systems. Sports Med 31(12):841–861
47. Christensen CC, Frey H, Foenstelien E, Aadland E, Refsum HE (1983) A critical evaluation of energy expenditure estimates based on individual O_2 consumption/heart rate curves and average daily heart rate. Am J Clin Nutr 37(3):468–472
48. Strath SJ, Swartz AM, Bassett DR Jr, O'Brien WL, King GA, Ainsworth BE (2000) Evaluation of heart rate as a method for assessing moderate intensity physical activity. Med Sci Sports Exerc 32(9 Suppl):S465–S470
49. Westerterp KR (2009) Assessment of physical activity: a critical appraisal. Eur J Appl Physiol 105(6):823–828
50. Hevesi P, Wille S, Pirkl G, Wehn N, Lukowicz P (2014) Monitoring household activities and user location with a cheap, unobtrusive thermal sensor array. In: ACM international joint conference on pervasive and ubiquitous computing, Seattle, USA, 13–17 Sept 2014
51. Han J, Bhanu B (2005) Human activity recognition in thermal infrared imagery. In: IEEE Computer society conference on computer vision and pattern recognition—workshops, San Diego, USA, 21–23 Sept 2005
52. Culhane K, O'connor M, D Lyons, Lyons G (2005) Accelerometers in rehabilitation medicine for older adults. Age Ageing 34(6):556–560
53. McGrath MJ, Scanaill CN (2014) Sensor technologies: healthcare, wellness and environmental applications. Apress, USA

54. Khan A, Hammerla N, Mellor S, Plötz T (2016) Optimising sampling rates for accelerometer-based human activity recognition. Pattern Recognit Lett 73:33–40

55. Lee J, Kim J (2016) Energy-efficient real-time human activity recognition on smart mobile devices. Mob Inf Syst 2016:1–12

56. Lyden K, Kozey SL, Staudenmeyer JW, Freedson PS (2011) A comprehensive evaluation of commonly used accelerometer energy expenditure and MET prediction equations. Eur J Appl Physiol 111(2):187–201

57. Swartz AM, Strath SJ, Bassett DR, O'Brien WL, King GA, Ainsworth BE (2000) Estimation of energy expenditure using CSA accelerometers at hip and wrist sites. Med Sci Sports Exerc 32(9 Suppl):S450–S456

58. Crouter SE, Kuffel E, Haas JD, Frongillo EA, Bassett DR Jr (2010) A refined 2-regression model for the actigraph accelerometer. Med Sci Sports Exerc 42(5):1029–1037

59. Freedson PS, Melanson E, Sirard J (1998) Calibration of the computer science and applications, Inc. accelerometer. Med Sci Sports Exerc 30(5):777–781

60. Hendelman D, Miller K, Baggett C, Debold E, Freedson P (2000) Validity of accelerometry for the assessment of moderate intensity physical activity in the field. Med Sci Sports Exerc 32(9 Suppl):S442–S449

61. Freedson P, Bowles HR, Troiano R, Haskell W (2012) Assessment of physical activity using wearable monitors: recommendations for monitor calibration and use in the field. Med Sci Sports Exerc 44(1 Suppl):S1–S4

62. Yang C-C, Hsu Y-L (2010) A review of accelerometry-based wearable motion detectors for physical activity monitoring. Sensors 10(8):7772–7788

63. Office of Diseases Prevention and Health Promotion (2008) Physical activity guidelines for Americans. https://health.gov/paguidelines/. Accessed Nov· 2012

64. Plasqui G, Westerterp KR (2007) Physical activity assessment with accelerometers: an evaluation against doubly labeled water. Obesity 15(10):2371–2379

65. Kim Y, Beets MW, Welk GJ (2012) Everything you wanted to know about selecting the "right" Actigraph accelerometer cut-points for youth, but…: a systematic review. J Sci Med Sport 15(4):311–321

66. Brage S, Westgate K, Franks PW, Stegle O, Wright A, Ekelund U, Wareham NJ (2015) Estimation of free-living energy expenditure by heart rate and movement sensing: a doubly-labelled water study. PLoS ONE 10(9):e0137206

67. Rothney MP, Brychta RJ, Meade NN, Chen KY, Buchowski MS (2010) Validation of the actigraph two-regression model for predicting energy expenditure. Med Sci Sports Exerc 42(9):1785–1792

68. Kuffel EE, Crouter SE, Haas JD, Frongillo EA, Bassett DR (2011) Validity of estimating minute-by-minute energy expenditure of continuous walking bouts by accelerometry. Int J Behav Nutr Phys Act. https://doi.org/10.1186/1479-5868-8-92

69. Kim Y, Crouter SE, Lee J-M, Dixon PM, Gaesser GA, Welk GJ (2016) Comparisons of prediction equations for estimating energy expenditure in youth. J Sci Med Sport 19(1):35–40

70. Strath SJ, Pfeiffer KA, Whitt-Glover MC (2012) Accelerometer use with children, older adults, and adults with functional limitations. Med Sci Sports Exerc 44(1 Suppl):S77–85

71. Stephens SK, Takken T, Esliger DW, Pullenayegum E, Beyene J, Tremblay MS, Schneiderman J, Biggar D, Longmuir P, McCrindle B (2016) Validation of accelerometer prediction equations in children with chronic disease. Pediatr Exerc Sci 28(1):117–132

72. Staudenmayer J, Pober D, Crouter S, Bassett D, Freedson P (2009) An artificial neural network to estimate physical activity energy expenditure and identify physical activity type from an accelerometer. J Appl Psychol 107(4):1300–1307

73. Zhang S, Rowlands AV, Murray P, Hurst TL (2012) Physical activity classification using the GENEA wrist-worn accelerometer. Med Sci Sports Exerc 44(4):742–748

74. Grünewälder S, Broekhuis F, Macdonald DW, Wilson AM, McNutt JW, Shawe-Taylor J, Hailes S (2012) Movement activity based classification of animal behaviour with an application to data from cheetah (Acinonyx jubatus). PLoS ONE 7(11):e49120

75. Pober DM, Staudenmayer J, Raphael C, Freedson PS (2006) Development of novel techniques to classify physical activity mode using accelerometers. Med Sci Sports Exerc 38(9):1626
76. Yang M, Zheng H, Wang H, McClean S, Hall J, Harris N (2012) A machine learning approach to assessing gait patterns for complex regional pain syndrome. Med Eng Phys 34(6):740–746
77. Arif M, Kattan A (2015) Physical activities monitoring using wearable acceleration sensors attached to the body. PLoS ONE 10(7):e0130851
78. Arif M, Kattan A, Ahamed SI (2017) Classification of physical activities using wearable sensors. Intell Autom Soft Co 23(1):21–30
79. Jensen U, Leutheuser H, Hofmann S, Schuepferling B, Suttner G, Seiler K, Kornhuber J, Eskofier BM (2015) A wearable real-time activity tracker. Biomed Eng Lett 5(2):147–157
80. Mathie M, Celler BG, Lovell NH, Coster A (2004) Classification of basic daily movements using a triaxial accelerometer. Med Biol Eng Comput 42(5):679–687
81. Ravi N, Dandekar N, Mysore P, Littman ML (2005) Activity recognition from accelerometer data. In: The 17th conference on Innovative applications of artificial intelligence, Pittsburgh, Pennsylbania, 9–13 Jul 2005
82. Kwapisz JR, Weiss GM, Moore SA (2011) Activity recognition using cell phone accelerometers. ACM SIGKDD Explor 12(2):74–82
83. Woznowski P, Kaleshi D, Oikonomou G, Craddock I (2016) Classification and suitability of sensing technologies for activity recognition. Comput Commun 89–90:34–50
84. Hammerla NY, Plötz T (2015) Let's (not) stick together: pairwise similarity biases cross-validation in activity recognition. In: Proceedings of the 2015 ACM international joint conference on pervasive and ubiquitous computing. ACM, pp 1041–1051
85. Alsheikh MA, Selim A, Niyato D, Doyle L, Lin S, Tan H-P (2015) Deep activity recognition models with triaxial accelerometers. https://arxiv.org/abs/1511.04664. Accessed Mar 2017
86. Hammerla NY, Halloran S, Ploetz T (2016) Deep, convolutional, and recurrent models for human activity recognition using wearables. https://arxiv.org/abs/1604.08880. Accessed Mar 2017
87. Hochreiter S, Schmidhuber J (1997) Long short-term memory. Neural Comput 9(8):1735–1780
88. Lu F, Wang D, Wu H, Xie W (2016) A multi-classifier combination method using SFFS algorithm for recognition of 19 human activities. In: Gervasi O et al (eds) Computational science and its applications—ICCSA 2016. ICCSA 2016. Lecture Notes in Computer Science, vol 9787. Springer, Cham
89. Lyden K, Keadle SK, Staudenmayer J, Freedson PS (2014) A method to estimate free-living active and sedentary behavior from an accelerometer. Med Sci Sports Exerc 46(2):386
90. Sasaki JE, Hickey AM, Staudenmayer JW, John D, Kent JA, Freedson PS (2016) Performance of activity classification algorithms in free-living older adults. Med Sci Sports Exerc 48(5):941–950
91. Hong J-H, Ramos J, Dey AK (2016) Toward personalized activity recognition systems with a semipopulation approach. IEEE Trans Human-Mach Syst 46(1):101–112
92. Butte NF, Ekelund U, Westerterp KR (2012) Assessing physical activity using wearable monitors: measures of physical activity. Med Sci Sports Exerc 44(1 Suppl):S5–S12
93. Matthew CE (2005) Calibration of accelerometer output for adults. Med Sci Sports Exerc 37(11 Suppl):S512–S522
94. Fried LP, Tangen CM, Walston J, Newman AB, Hirsch C, Gottdiener J, Seeman T, Tracy R, Kop WJ, Burke G (2001) Frailty in older adults evidence for a phenotype. J Gerontol A Biol Sci Med Sci 56(3):M146–M157
95. Castell M-V, Sánchez M, Julián R, Queipo R, Martín S, Otero Á (2013) Frailty prevalence and slow walking speed in persons age 65 and older: implications for primary care. BMC Fam Pract 14(1):86. https://doi.org/10.1186/1471-2296-14-86
96. Storti KL, Pettee KK, Brach JS, Talkowski JB, Richardson CR, Kriska AM (2008) Gait speed and step-count monitor accuracy in community-dwelling older adults. Med Sci Sports Exerc 40(1):59–64

97. Yoneyama M, Kurihara Y, Watanabe K, Mitoma H (2014) Accelerometry-based gait analysis and its application to parkinson's disease assessment—part 1: detection of stride event. IEEE Trans Neural Syst Rehabil Eng 22(3):613–622

98. Marschollek M, Goevercin M, Wolf K-H, Song B, Gietzelt M, Haux R, Steinhagen-Thiessen E (2008) A performance comparison of accelerometry-based step detection algorithms on a large, non-laboratory sample of healthy and mobility-impaired persons. In: 30th Annual international conference of the IEEE engineering in medicine and biology society. Conf Proc IEEE Eng Med Biol Soc, pp 1319–1322

99. Fortune E, Lugade V, Morrow M, Kaufman K (2014) Validity of using tri-axial accelerometers to measure human movement–Part II: step counts at a wide range of gait velocities. Med Eng Phys 36(6):659–669

100. Resnick B, Nahm E-S, Orwig D, Zimmerman SS, Magaziner J (2001) Measurement of activity in older adults: reliability and validity of the step activity monitor. J Nurs Meas 9(3):275–290

101. Haeuber E, Shaughnessy M, Forrester LW, Coleman KL, Macko RF (2004) Accelerometer monitoring of home-and community-based ambulatory activity after stroke. Arch Phys Med Rehabil 85(12):1997–2001

102. Soaz C, Diepold K (2016) Step detection and parameterization for gait assessment using a single waist-worn accelerometer. IEEE Trans Biomed Eng 63(5):933–942

103. Rietveld P, Daniel V (2004) Determinants of bicycle use: do municipal policies matter? Transp Res A 38(7):531–550

104. Long X, Yin B, Aarts RM (2009) Single-accelerometer-based daily physical activity classification. In: Annual international conference in medicine and biology society. Conf Proc IEEE Eng Med Biol Soc, pp 6107–6110

105. Alshurafa N, Xu W, Liu JJ, Huang M-C, Mortazavi B, Roberts CK, Sarrafzadeh M (2014) Designing a robust activity recognition framework for health and exergaming using wearable sensors. IEEE J Biomed Health Inform 18(5):1636–1646

106. Bonomi AG, Goris A, Yin B, Westerterp KR (2009) Detection of type, duration, and intensity of physical activity using an accelerometer. Med Sci Sports Exerc 41(9):1770–1777

107. Fahim M, Fatima I, Lee S, Park Y-T (2013) EFM: evolutionary fuzzy model for dynamic activities recognition using a smartphone accelerometer. Appl intell 39(3):475–488

108. Attal F, Mohammed S, Dedabrishvili M, Chamroukhi F, Oukhellou L, Amirat Y (2015) Physical human activity recognition using wearable sensors. Sensors 15(12):31314–31338

109. Xu W, Zhang M, Sawchuk AA, Sarrafzadeh M (2012) Robust human activity and sensor location corecognition via sparse signal representation. IEEE Trans Biomed Eng 59(11):3169–3176

110. Gemperle F, Kasabach C, Stivoric J, Bauer M, Martin R (1998) Design for wearability. In: 2nd International symposium on wearable computers, Pittsburgh, USA, 19–20 Oct 1998

111. Hill C (2015) Wearables–the future of biometric technology? Biometric Technol Today 8:5–9

112. Najafi B, Aminian K, Paraschiv-Ionescu A, Loew F, Bula CJ, Robert P (2003) Ambulatory system for human motion analysis using a kinematic sensor: monitoring of daily physical activity in the elderly. IEEE Trans Biomed Eng 50(6):711–723

113. Lindemann U, Hock A, Stuber M, Keck W, Becker C (2005) Evaluation of a fall detector based on accelerometers: a pilot study. Med Biol Eng Comput 43(5):548–551

114. Olivares A, Olivares G, Mula F, Górriz J, Ramírez J (2011) Wagyromag: wireless sensor network for monitoring and processing human body movement in healthcare applications. J Syst Architect 57(10):905–915

115. Fitbit (2016) Fitbit Chrage HR(TM) https://www.fitbit.com/uk/chargehr. Accessed Mar 2016

116. Microsoft (2016) Microsoft-Band. https://www.microsoft.com/microsoft-band/en-gb. Accessed Jan 2018

117. Jawbone (2016) UP2. https://jawbone.com/store/buy/up2. Accessed Nov 2017

118. Wearable Nike FuelBand: The rise and fall of the wearable that started it all. http://www.wareable.com/nike/not-so-happy-birthday-nike-fuelband-2351. Accessed Jan 2018

119. Prest C, Hoellwarth QC (2014) Sports monitoring system for headphones, earbuds and/or headsets. US Patent 8655004B2, 16 Nov 2007

120. Jabra (2015) JABRA SPORT COACH. http://www.jabra.co.uk/sports-headphones/jabra-spo
     rt-coach-wireless. Accessed Jan 2018
121. Menz HB, Lord SR, Fitzpatrick RC (2003) Acceleration patterns of the head and pelvis when
     walking are associated with risk of falling in community-dwelling older people. J Gerontol
     A Biol Sci Med Sci 58(5):M446–M452
122. McClusky M (2009) The Nike experiment: how the shoe giant unleashed the power of personal
     metrics. https://www.wired.com/2009/06/lbnp-nike/. Accessed Dec 2017
123. Dittmar A, Lymberis (2005) A Smart clothes and associated wearable devices for biomedical
     ambulatory monitoring. In: The 13th International conference on solid-state sensors, actuators
     and microsystems, Seoul, Korea, 5–9 Jun 2005
124. Patel S, Park H, Bonato P, Chan L, Rodgers M (2012) A review of wearable sensors and
     systems with application in rehabilitation. J Neuroeng Rehabil 9:21. https://doi.org/10.1186/
     1743-0003-9-21
125. Poon CC, Liu Q, Gao H, Lin W-H, Zhang Y-T (2011) Wearable intelligent systems for e-health.
     JCSE 5(3):246–256
126. Huberty J, Ehlers DK, Kurka J, Ainsworth B, Buman M (2015) Feasibility of three wearable
     sensors for 24 hour monitoring in middle-aged women. BMC Womens Health 15:55. https://
     doi.org/10.1186/s12905-015-0212-3
127. Ellis K, Kerr J, Godbole S, Staudenmayer J, Lanckriet G (2016) Hip and wrist accelerometer
     algorithms for free-living behavior classification. Med Sci Sports Exerc 48(5):933–940
128. McFedries P (2014) The inescapability of ambient computing; always-listening, always-
     watching computers want to help—maybe too much. In: IEEE Spectrum. http://spectrum.
     ieee.org/computing/it/the-inescapability-of-ambient-computing. Accessed Sept 2017
129. Ju AL, Spasojevic M (2015) Smart jewelry: the future of mobile user interfaces. In: Workshop
     on future mobile user interfaces, Florence, Italy, 18 May 2015
130. Oura (2018) Oura Ring. https://ouraring.com/. Accessed Mar 2018
131. Silva AS, Salazar AJ, Correia MV, Borges CM (2011) WIMU: wearable inertial monitoring
     unit-A MEMS-based device for swimming performance analysis. https://paginas.fe.up.pt/~d
     ee08011/files/Download/BIODEVICES2011.pdf. Accessed Dec 2017
132. Paradiso R, Gemignani A, Scilingo E, De Rossi D (2003) Knitted bioclothes for cardiopul-
     monary monitoring. In: Proceedings of the 25th annual international conference of the ieee
     engineering in medicine and biology society, Cancun, Mexico, 17–21 Sept 2003
133. Di Rienzo M, Rizzo F, Parati G, Brambilla G, Ferratini M, Castiglioni P (2005) MagIC
     system: A new textile-based wearable device for biological signal monitoring. Applicability
     in daily life and clinical setting. In: Proceedings of the 2005 IEEE Engineering in Medicine
     and Biology 27th Annual Conference, Shanghai, China, 1–4 Sept 2005. Conf Proc IEEE Eng
     Med Biol Soc 7:7167–7169
134. Niazmand K, Neuhaeuser J, Lueth TC (2012) A washable smart shirt for the measurement of
     activity in every-day life. In: Wichert R, Eberhardt B (eds) Ambient assisted living. Advanced
     technologies and societal change. Springer, Heidelbert, pp 333–345
135. Pirotte F, Klefstad-Sillonville F (2006) MERMOTH: medical remote monitoring of clothes.
     https://cordis.europa.eu/project/rcn/72234_en.html. Accessed Jan 2018
136. Noury N, Dittmar A, Corroy C, Baghai R, Weber J, Blanc D, Klefstat F, Blinovska A, Vaysse S,
     Comet B (2004) VTAMN-A smart clothe for ambulatory remote monitoring of physiological
     parameters and activity. In: Proceedings of 26th annual IEEE International Conference on
     Engineering In Medicine and Biology Society, San Francisco, USA, 1–5 Sept 2004. Conf
     Proc IEEE Eng Med Biol Soc, pp 3266–3269
137. Pacelli M, Loriga G, Taccini N, Paradiso R (2006) Sensing fabrics for monitoring physiological
     and biomechanical variables: E-textile solutions. In: Proceedings of the 3rd IEEE-EMBS,
     international summer school and symposium on medical devices and biosensors, Boston,
     USA, 4–6 Sept 2006
138. Altini M, Penders J, Vullers R, Amft O (2015) Estimating energy expenditure using body-worn
     accelerometers: a comparison of methods, sensors number and positioning. IEEE J Biomed
     Health Inform 19(1):219–226

139. Cleland I, Kikhia B, Nugent C, Boytsov A, Hallberg J, Synnes K, McClean S, Finlay D (2013) Optimal placement of accelerometers for the detection of everyday activities. Sensors 13(7):9183–9200

140. Mathie MJ, Coster AC, Lovell NH, Celler BG (2004) Accelerometry: providing an integrated, practical method for long-term, ambulatory monitoring of human movement. Physiol Meas 25(2):R1–R20

141. Zhang JH, Macfarlane DJ, Sobko T (2016) Feasibility of a chest-worn accelerometer for physical activity measurement. J Sci Med Sport 19(12):1015–1019

142. Gjoreski M, Gjoreski H, Luštrek M, Gams M (2016) How accurately can your wrist device recognize daily activities and detect falls? Sensors 16(6). https://doi.org/10.3390/s16060800

143. Oshin TO, Poslad S (2013) ERSP: An energy-efficient real-time smartphone pedometer. In: 2013 IEEE International conference on systems, man, and cybernetics, Manchester, UK, 13–16 Oct 2013

144. Kammoun S, Pothin J-B, Cousin J-C (2015) An efficient fuzzy logic step detection algorithm for unconstrained smartphones. In: 2015 IEEE 26th Annual international symposium on personal, indoor, and mobile radio communications (PIMRC): services, applications and business, Hong Kong, China, 30 Aug–2 Sept 2015

145. H-h Lee, Choi S, M-j Lee (2015) Step detection robust against the dynamics of smartphones. Sensors 15(9):27230–27250

146. Kunze K, Lukowicz P, Junker H, Tröster G (2005) Where Am I: Recognizing on-body positions of wearable sensors. In: Strang T, Linnhoff-Popien C (eds) Location- and Context-Awareness. LoCA 2005. Lecture Notes in Computer Science, vol 3479. Springer, Berlin, Heidelberg

147. Amini N, Sarrafzadeh M, Vahdatpour A, Xu W (2011) Accelerometer-based on-body sensor localization for health and medical monitoring applications. Pervasive Mobile Comput 7(6):746–760

148. Mannini A, Sabatini AM, Intille SS (2015) Accelerometry-based recognition of the placement sites of a wearable sensor. Pervasive Mobile Comput 21:62–74

149. Vahdatpour A, Amini N, Sarrafzadeh M (2011) On-body device localization for health and medical monitoring applications. In: 2011 IEEE International conference on pervasive computing and communications (PerCom), Seattle, USA, 21–25 Mar 2011

150. del Rosario MB, Redmond SJ, Lovell NH (2015) Tracking the evolution of smartphone sensing for monitoring human movement. Sensors 15(8):18901–18933

151. Zhang Z-Q, Yang G-Z (2015) Micromagnetometer calibration for accurate orientation estimation. IEEE Trans Biomed Eng 62(2):553–560

152. Kok M, Hol JD, Schön TB, Gustafsson F, Luinge H (2012) Calibration of a magnetometer in combination with inertial sensors. In: 15th International conference on information fusion (FUSION), Singapore, 9–12 July 2012

153. Alonso R, Shuster MD (2002) TWOSTEP: A fast robust algorithm for attitude-independent magnetometer-bias determination. J Astronaut Sci 50(4):433–452

154. Gebre-Egziabher D, Elkaim GH, David Powell J, Parkinson BW (2006) Calibration of strapdown magnetometers in magnetic field domain. J Astronaut Sci 19(2):87–102

155. Hellénius M-L, Sundberg CJ (2011) Physical activity as medicine: time to translate evidence into clinical practice. Brit J Sport Med 45(3):158–158

156. Ganesan AN, Louise J, Horsfall M, Bilsborough SA, Hendriks J, McGavigan AD, Selvanayagam JB, Chew DP (2016) International mobile-health intervention on physical activity, sitting, and weight: The Stepathlon Cardiovascular Health Study. J Am Coll Cardiol 67(21):2453–2463

157. Mateo GF, Granado-Font E, Ferré-Grau C, Montaña-Carreras X (2015) Mobile phone apps to promote weight loss and increase physical activity: A systematic review and meta-analysis. J Med Internet Res 17(11). https://dio.org/10.2196/jmir.4836

158. WHO (2014) mHealth: New horizons for health through mobile technologies: Second global survey on eHealth. http://www.who.int/goe/publications/goe_mhealth_web.pdf. Accessed Feb 2018

159. Martin SS, Feldman DI, Blumenthal RS, Jones SR, Post WS, McKibben RA, Michos ED, Ndumele CE, Ratchford EV, Coresh J (2015) mActive: a randomized clinical trial of an automated mHealth intervention for physical activity promotion. J Am Heart Assoc 4(11):e002239

160. Bamidis P, Vivas A, Styliadis C, Frantzidis C, Klados M, Schlee W, Siountas A, Papageorgiou S (2014) A review of physical and cognitive interventions in aging. Neurosci Biobehav Rev 44:206–220

161. Baranowski T, Baranowski J, O'Connor T, Lu AS, Thompson D (2012) Is enhanced physical activity possible using active videogames? Games Health J 1(3):228–232

162. Maillot P, Perrot A, Hartley A (2012) Effects of interactive physical-activity video-game training on physical and cognitive function in older adults. Psychol Aging 27(3):589

163. de Bruin PDE, Schoene D, Pichierri G, Smith ST (2010) Use of virtual reality technique for the training of motor control in the elderly. Zeitschrift für Gerontologie und Geriatrie 43(4):229–234

164. Bisson E, Contant B, Sveistrup H, Lajoie Y (2007) Functional balance and dual-task reaction times in older adults are improved by virtual reality and biofeedback training. Cyberpsychol Behav 10(1):16–23

165. Rendon AA, Lohman EB, Thorpe D, Johnson EG, Medina E, Bradley B (2012) The effect of virtual reality gaming on dynamic balance in older adults. Age Ageing 41(4):549–552

166. Molina KI, Ricci NA, de Moraes SA, Perracini MR (2014) Virtual reality using games for improving physical functioning in older adults: a systematic review. J Neuroeng Rehabil 11:156. https://doi.org/10.1186/1743-0003-11-156

167. Van Diest M, Stegenga J, Wörtche H, Verkerke G, Postema K, Lamoth C (2016) Exergames for unsupervised balance training at home: a pilot study in healthy older adults. Gait Posture 44:161–167

168. Van Diest M, Lamoth CJ, Stegenga J, Verkerke GJ, Postema K (2013) Exergaming for balance training of elderly: state of the art and future developments. J Neuroeng Rehabil 10(1):101. https://doi.org/10.1186/1743-0003-10-101

169. Hoffman HG, Richards T, Coda B, Richards A, Sharar SR (2003) The illusion of presence in immersive virtual reality during an fMRI brain scan. Cyberpsychol Behav 6(2):127–131

170. Viskaal-van Dongen M, Kok FJ, de Graaf C (2011) Eating rate of commonly consumed foods promotes food and energy intake. Appetite 56(1):25–31

171. Ohkuma T, Hirakawa Y, Nakamura U, Kiyohara Y, Kitazono T, Ninomiya T (2015) Association between eating rate and obesity: a systematic review and meta-analysis. Int J Obesity 39(11):1589–1596

172. Saneei P, Esmaillzadeh A, Keshteli AH, Feizi A, Feinle-Bisset C, Adibi P (2016) Patterns of dietary habits in relation to obesity in Iranian adults. Eur J Nutr 55(2):713–728

173. Tanihara S, Imatoh T, Miyazaki M, Babazono A, Momose Y, Baba M, Uryu Y, Une H (2011) Retrospective longitudinal study on the relationship between 8-year weight change and current eating speed. Appetite 57(1):179–183

174. Palladino-Davis A, Mendez B, Fisichella P, Davis C (2015) Dietary habits and esophageal cancer. Dis Esophagus 28(1):59–67

175. Bertuccio P, Rosato V, Andreano A, Ferraroni M, Decarli A, Edefonti V, La Vecchia C (2013) Dietary patterns and gastric cancer risk: a systematic review and meta-analysis. Ann Oncol 24(6):1450–1458

176. Albuquerque RC, Baltar VT, Marchioni DM (2014) Breast cancer and dietary patterns: a systematic review. Nutr Rev 72(1):1–17

177. Vance TM, Su J, Fontham ET, Koo SI, Chun OK (2013) Dietary antioxidants and prostate cancer: a review. Nutr Cancer 65(6):793–801

178. Aune D, Norat T, Romundstad P, Vatten LJ (2013) Dairy products and the risk of type 2 diabetes: a systematic review and dose-response meta-analysis of cohort studies. Am J Clin Nutr 98(4):1066–1083

179. Gemming L, Utter J, Mhurchu CN (2015) Image-assisted dietary assessment: a systematic review of the evidence. J Acad Nutr Diet 115(1):64–77

180. Hermsen S, Frost JH, Robinson E, Higgs S, Mars M, Hermans RC (2016) Evaluation of a smart fork to decelerate eating rate. J Acad Nutr Diet 116(7):1066–1068

181. Zhou B, Cheng J, Lukowicz P, Reiss A, Amft O (2015) Monitoring dietary behavior with a smart dining tray. IEEE Pervasive Comput 14(4):46–56

182. Zhou B, Cheng J, Sundholm M, Reiss A, Huang W, Amft O, Lukowicz P (2015) Smart table surface: a novel approach to pervasive dining monitoring. In: IEEE International conference on pervasive computing and communications (PerCom), St. Louis, USA, 23–27 Mar 2015

183. Luo S, Xia H, Gao Y, Jin JS, Athauda R (2008) Smart fridges with multimedia capability for better nutrition and health. In: international symposium on ubiquitous multimedia computing, Hobart, Australia, 13–15 Oct 2008

184. Luo S, Jin J, Li J (2009) A smart fridge with an ability to enhance health and enable better nutrition. Int J Multimedia Ubiquitous Eng 4(2):66–80

185. Gu H, Wang D (2009) A content-aware fridge based on RFID in smart home for home-healthcare. In: 11th International conference on advanced communication technology, Gangwon-Do, South Korea, 15–18 Feb 2009

186. Yam KL, Takhistov PT, Miltz J (2005) Intelligent packaging: concepts and applications. J Food Sci 70(1):R1–R10

187. Prestwic E (2016) Naraffar, Unmanned Swedish Grocery Store, Open 24 Hours. http://www.huffingtonpost.ca/2016/03/16/naraffar-sweden-unmanned-grocery-store_n_9480270.html. Accessed Aug 2016

188. Boulos MNK, Yassine A, Shirmohammadi S, Namahoot CS, Brückner M (2015) Towards an "Internet of Food": food ontologies for the internet of things. Future Internet 7(4):372–392

189. Arem H, Moore SC, Patel A, Hartge P, de Gonzalez AB, Visvanathan K, Campbell PT, Freedman M, Weiderpass E, Adami HO (2015) Leisure time physical activity and mortality: a detailed pooled analysis of the dose-response relationship. JAMA Intern Med 175(6):959–967

190. Smith SC, Collins A, Ferrari R, Holmes DR, Logstrup S, McGhie DV, Ralston J, Sacco RL, Stam H, Taubert K (2012) Our time: a call to save preventable death from cardiovascular disease (heart disease and stroke). Eur Heart J 33(23):2910–2916

191. Vorrink S (2016) eHealth to stimulate physical activity in patients with chronic obstructive pulmonary disease. Dissertation, University of Applied Sciences Utrecht

192. Varghese T, Schultz WM, McCue AA, Lambert CT, Sandesara PB, Eapen DJ, Gordon NF, Franklin BA, Sperling LS (2016) Physical activity in the prevention of coronary heart disease: implications for the clinician. Heart (British Cardiac Society). https://doi.org/10.1136/heartjnl-2015-308773

193. Intwala S, Balady GJ (2015) Physical activity in the prevention of heart failure: another step forward. Circulation. https://doi.org/10.1161/CIRCULATIONAHA.115.018831

194. Lloyd-Jones DM, Hong Y, Labarthe D, Mozaffarian D, Appel LJ, Van Horn L, Greenlund K, Daniels S, Nichol G, Tomaselli GF (2010) Defining and setting national goals for cardiovascular health promotion and disease reduction the American Heart Association's Strategic Impact Goal through 2020 and beyond. Circulation 121(4):586–613

195. Kokkinos P (2012) Physical activity, health benefits, and mortality risk. ISRN cardiology. https://doi.org/10.5402/2012/718789

196. Mora S, Redberg RF, Cui Y, Whiteman MK, Flaws JA, Sharrett AR, Blumenthal RS (2003) Ability of exercise testing to predict cardiovascular and all-cause death in asymptomatic women: a 20-year follow-up of the lipid research clinics prevalence study. JAMA 290(12):1600–1607

197. Gulati M, Pandey DK, Arnsdorf MF, Lauderdale DS, Thisted RA, Wicklund RH, Al-Hani AJ, Black HR (2003) Exercise capacity and the risk of death in women the St James Women take heart project. Circulation 108(13):1554–1559

198. Myers J, Prakash M, Froelicher V, Do D, Partington S, Atwood JE (2002) Exercise capacity and mortality among men referred for exercise testing. New Engl J Med 346(11):793–801

199. Kokkinos P, Manolis A, Pittaras A, Doumas M, Giannelou A, Panagiotakos DB, Faselis C, Narayan P, Singh S, Myers J (2009) Exercise capacity and mortality in hypertensive men with and without additional risk factors. Hypertension 53(3):494–499

200. Blair SN, Kohl HW, Barlow CE, Gibbons LW (1991) Physical fitness and all-cause mortality in hypertensive men. Ann Med 23(3):307–312
201. Faselis C, Doumas M, Panagiotakos D, Kheirbek R, Korshak L, Manolis A, Pittaras A, Tsioufis C, Papademetriou V, Fletcher R (2012) Body mass index, exercise capacity, and mortality risk in male veterans with hypertension. Am J Hypertens 25(4):444–450
202. Helmrich SP, Ragland DR, Leung RW, Paffenbarger RS Jr (1991) Physical activity and reduced occurrence of non-insulin-dependent diabetes mellitus. New Engl J Med 325(3):147–152
203. Manson JE, Nathan DM, Krolewski AS, Stampfer MJ, Willett WC, Hennekens CH (1992) A prospective study of exercise and incidence of diabetes among US male physicians. JAMA 268(1):63–67
204. Hu FB, Sigal RJ, Rich-Edwards JW, Colditz GA, Solomon CG, Willett WC, Speizer FE, Manson JE (1999) Walking compared with vigorous physical activity and risk of type 2 diabetes in women: a prospective study. JAMA 282(15):1433–1439
205. Honda T, Kuwahara K, Nakagawa T, Yamamoto S, Hayashi T, Mizoue T (2015) Leisure-time, occupational, and commuting physical activity and risk of type 2 diabetes in Japanese workers: a cohort study. BMC Public Health. https://doi.org/10.1186/s12966-015-0283-4
206. Rasmussen MG, Grøntved A, Blond K, Overvad K, Tjønneland A, Jensen MK, Østergaard L (2016) Associations between recreational and commuter cycling, changes in cycling, and type 2 diabetes risk: a cohort study of Danish men and women. PLoS Med 13(7):e1002076
207. Lecomte P, Cacès E, Born C, Chabrolle C, Lasfargues G, Halimi J-M, Tichet J (2007) Five-year predictive factors of type 2 diabetes in men with impaired fasting glucose. Diab Metab 33(2):140–147
208. Lynch J, Helmrich SP, Lakka TA, Kaplan GA, Cohen RD, Salonen R, Salonen JT (1996) Moderately intense physical activities and high levels of cardiorespiratory fitness reduce the risk of non-insulin-dependent diabetes mellitus in middle-aged men. Arch Intern Med 156(12):1307–1314
209. Villegas R, Shu X-O, Li H, Yang G, Matthews CE, Leitzmann M, Li Q, Cai H, Gao Y-T, Zheng W (2006) Physical activity and the incidence of type 2 diabetes in the Shanghai women's health study. Int J Epidemiol 35(6):1553–1562
210. Laaksonen MA, Knekt P, Rissanen H, Härkänen T, Virtala E, Marniemi J, Aromaa A, Heliövaara M, Reunanen A (2010) The relative importance of modifiable potential risk factors of type 2 diabetes: a meta-analysis of two cohorts. Eur J Epidemiol 25(2):115–124
211. Group DPPR (2002) Reduction in the incidence of type 2 diabetes with lifestyle intervention or metformin. N Engl J Med (346)(6):393–403
212. Group DPPR (2004) Achieving weight and activity goals among diabetes prevention program lifestyle participants. Obes Res 12(9):1426
213. Vähäsarja K, Kasila K, Kettunen T, Rintala P, Salmela S, Poskiparta M (2015) 'I saw what the future direction would be…': experiences of diabetes risk and physical activity after diabetes screening. Brit J Health Psych 20(1):172–193
214. Wareham NJ, Brage S, Franks PW, Abbott RA (2005) Physical Activity and Insulin Resistance. In: Kumar S, O'Rahilly S (eds) Insulin resistance: Insulin action and its disturbances in disease. Wiley & Sons, USA
215. Aune D, Norat T, Leitzmann M, Tonstad S, Vatten LJ (2015) Physical activity and the risk of type 2 diabetes: a systematic review and dose–response meta-analysis. Eur J Epidemiol 30(7):529–542
216. Joseph JJ, Echouffo-Tcheugui JB, Golden SH, Chen H, Jenny NS, Carnethon MR, Jacobs D, Burke GL, Vaidya D, Ouyang P (2016) Physical activity, sedentary behaviors and the incidence of type 2 diabetes mellitus: the Multi-Ethnic Study of Atherosclerosis (MESA). BMJ Open Diabetes Res Care 4(1):e000185
217. Sigal RJ, Armstrong MJ, Colby P, Kenny GP, Plotnikoff RC, Reichert SM, Riddell MC (2013) Physical activity and diabetes. Can J Diabetes 37:S40–S44
218. Wadén J, Tikkanen HK, Forsblom C, Harjutsalo V, Thorn LM, Saraheimo M, Tolonen N, Rosengård-Bärlund M, Gordin D, Tikkanen HO (2015) Leisure-time physical activity and development and progression of diabetic nephropathy in type 1 diabetes: the FinnDiane Study. Diabetologia 58(5):929–936

219. Russo LM, Nobles C, Ertel KA, Chasan-Taber L, Whitcomb BW (2015) Physical activity interventions in pregnancy and risk of gestational diabetes mellitus: a systematic review and meta-analysis. Obst Gynecol 125(3):576–582

220. Mathers CD, Loncar D (2005) Updated projections of global mortality and burden of disease, 2002–2030: data sources, methods and results. http://www.who.int/healthinfo/statistics/bod_projections2030_paper.pdf

221. Wiles NJ, Haase AM, Lawlor DA, Ness A, Lewis G (2012) Physical activity and depression in adolescents: cross-sectional findings from the ALSPAC cohort. Soc Psych Psych Epid 47(7):1023–1033

222. Babiss LA, Gangwisch JE (2009) Sports participation as a protective factor against depression and suicidal ideation in adolescents as mediated by self-esteem and social support. J Dev Behav Pediatr 30(5):376–384

223. Hong X, Li J, Xu F, Tse LA, Liang Y, Wang Z, Yu IT-s, Griffiths S (2009) Physical activity inversely associated with the presence of depression among urban adolescents in regional China. BMC Public Health 9(148). https://doi.org/10.1186/1471-2458-9-148

224. Eyre HA, Papps E, Baune BT (2015) Treating depression and depression-like behavior with physical activity: an immune perspective. Front Psychiatry 4:3. https://doi.org/10.3389/fpsyt.2013.00003

225. Göhner W, Dietsche C, Fuchs R (2015) Increasing physical activity in patients with mental illness—a randomized controlled trial. Patient Educ Couns 98(11):1385–1392

226. Knöchel C, Oertel-Knöchel V, O'Dwyer L, Prvulovic D, Alves G, Kollmann B, Hampel H (2012) Cognitive and behavioural effects of physical exercise in psychiatric patients. Prog Neurobiol 96(1):46–68

227. Spruit A, Assink M, van Vugt E, van der Put C, Stams GJ (2016) The effects of physical activity interventions on psychosocial outcomes in adolescents: a meta-analytic review. Clin Psychol Rev 45:56–71

228. Lindegård A, Jonsdottir IH, Börjesson M, Lindwall M, Gerber M (2015) Changes in mental health in compliers and non-compliers with physical activity recommendations in patients with stress-related exhaustion. BMC psychiatry 15:272. https://doi.org/10.1186/s12888-015-0642-3

229. Öhman H, Savikko N, Strandberg T, Kautiainen H, Raivio M, Laakkonen M-L, Tilvis R, Pitkälä KH (2016) Effects of exercise on functional performance and fall rate in subjects with mild or advanced Alzheimer's disease: secondary analyses of a randomized controlled study. Dement Geriatr Cogn 41(3–4):233–241

230. Burton E, Cavalheri V, Adams R, Browne CO, Bovery-Spencer P, Fenton AM, Campbell BW, Hill KD (2015) Effectiveness of exercise programs to reduce falls in older people with dementia living in the community: a systematic review and meta-analysis. Clin Interv Aging 10:421–434

231. Chan WC, Yeung JWF, Wong CSM, Lam LCW, Chung KF, Luk JKH, Lee JSW, Law ACK (2015) Efficacy of physical exercise in preventing falls in older adults with cognitive impairment: a systematic review and meta-analysis. J Am Med Dir Assoc 16(2):149–154

232. Alzheimer's Disease International (2014) Alzheimer's Disease International Dementia Statistics. http://www.alz.co.uk/research/statistics. Accessed Apr 2016

233. Sowa M, Meulenbroek R (2012) Effects of physical exercise on autism spectrum disorders: a meta-analysis. Res Autism Spect Dis 6(1):46–57

234. Memari A, Ghaheri B, Ziaee V, Kordi R, Hafizi S, Moshayedi P (2013) Physical activity in children and adolescents with autism assessed by triaxial accelerometry. Pediatr Obes 8(2):150–158

235. Young S (2016) Exercise effects in individuals with autism spectrum disorder: a short review. Autism Open Access 6(3):1000180

236. Lorenz EC, Amer H, Dean PG, Stegall MD, Cosio FG, Cheville AL (2015) Adherence to a pedometer-based physical activity intervention following kidney transplant and impact on metabolic parameters. Clin Transplant 29(6):560–568

237. Leuenberger K, Gonzenbach R, Wachter S, Luft A, Gassert R (2016) A method to qualitatively assess arm use in stroke survivors in the home environment. Med Biol Eng Comput 55(1):141–150

238. West J, Hippisley-Cox J, Coupland CA, Price G, Groom L, Kendrick D, Webber E (2004) Do rates of hospital admission for falls and hip fracture in elderly people vary by socio-economic status? Public Health 118(8):576–581

239. O'Loughlin JL, Robitaille Y, Boivin J-F, Suissa S (1993) Incidence of and risk factors for falls and injurious falls among the community-dwelling elderly. Am J Epidemiol 137(3):342–354

240. Gill T, Taylor AW, Pengelly A (2005) A population-based survey of factors relating to the prevalence of falls in older people. Gerontology 51(5):340–345

241. De Rekeneire N, Visser M, Peila R, Nevitt MC, Cauley JA, Tylavsky FA, Simonsick EM, Harris TB (2003) Is a fall just a fall: correlates of falling in healthy older persons. The health, aging and body composition study. J Am Geriatr Soc 51(6):841–846

242. Tinetti ME, Baker DI, King M, Gottschalk M, Murphy TE, Acampora D, Carlin BP, Leo-Summers L, Allore HG (2008) Effect of dissemination of evidence in reducing injuries from falls. New Engl J Med 359(3):252–261

243. Chenore T, Gray DP, Forrer J, Wright C, Evans P (2013) Emergency hospital admissions for the elderly: insights from the Devon Predictive Model. J Pub Health 35(4):616–623

244. Shumway-Cook A, Baldwin M, Polissar NL, Gruber W (1997) Predicting the probability for falls in community-dwelling older adults. Phys Ther 77(8):812–819

245. Kim S-B, Zingmond DS, Keeler EB, Jennings LA, Wenger NS, Reuben DB, Ganz DA (2016) Development of an algorithm to identify fall-related injuries and costs in Medicare data. Inj Epidemiol 3:1. https://doi.org/10.1186/s40621-015-0066-z

246. Office for National Statistics (2015) National Population Projections: 2014-based Statistical Bulletin. https://www.ons.gov.uk/peoplepopulationandcommunity/populationandmigration/populationprojections/bulletins/nationalpopulationprojections/2015-10-29. Accessed Dec 2017

247. European Commission (2012) The 2012 Ageing Report. Economic and budgetary projections for the 27 EU Member States (2010–2060). http://ec.europa.eu/economy_finance/publications/european_economy/2012/pdf/ee-2012-2_en.pdf. Accessed Dec 2017

248. Malnick E (2014) 10 per cent rise in number of people living alone. Telegraph Media Group. http://www.telegraph.co.uk/news/health/elder/11299527/10-per-cent-rise-in-number-of-people-living-alone.html. Accessed Dec 2017

249. Fairbanks M, Davis M, Jacob T, Sanchez M, Hugo B (2016) Epidemiology of Hip Fractures, a Retrospective Review. https://digitalcommons.hsc.unt.edu/rad/RAD16/CommunityMedicine/2/. Accessed Dec 2017

250. Tajeu GS, Delzell E, Smith W, Arora T, Curtis JR, Saag KG, Morrisey MA, Yun H, Kilgore ML (2013) Death, debility, and destitution following hip fracture. J Gerontol A Biol Sci Med Sci 69(3):346–353

251. Fletcher PC, Hirdes JP (2002) Risk factors for falling among community-based seniors using home care services. J Gerontol A Biol Sci Med Sci 57(8):M504–M510

252. Hendrich A, Nyhuis A, Kippenbrock T, Soja ME (1995) Hospital falls: development of a predictive model for clinical practice. Appl Nurs Res 8(3):129–139

253. Stevens JA, Corso PS, Finkelstein EA, Miller TR (2006) The costs of fatal and non-fatal falls among older adults. Inj Prev 12(5):290–295

254. Department of Health and Ageing of Australian Government (2004) An analysis of research on preventing falls and falls injury in older people: Community, residential care and hospital settings. https://www.health.gov.au/internet/main/publishing.nsf/Content/14D0B87F9C15C1E8CA257BF0001DC537/$File/falls_community.pdf. Accessed May 2017

255. Tinetti ME, Liu W-L, Claus EB (1993) Predictors and prognosis of inability to get up after falls among elderly persons. JAMA 269(1):65–70

256. Lai DTH, Palaniswami M, Begg R (2016) Healthcare sensor networks: challenges toward practical implementation. CRC Press, USA

257. Rubenstein LZ, Josephson KR (2002) The epidemiology of falls and syncope. Clin Geriatr Med 18(2):141–158

258. Williams G, Doughty K, Cameron K, Bradley D (1998) A smart fall and activity monitor for telecare applications. In: Proceedings of the 20th annual international conference of the IEEE engineering in medicine and biology society, Hong Kong, China, 29 Oct–1 Nov 1998

259. Sposaro F, Tyson G (2009) iFall: an android application for fall monitoring and response. In: Annual international conference of the IEEE engineering in medicine and biology society, Minnesota, USA, 2–6 Sept 2009

260. Kansiz AO, Guvensan MA, Turkmen HI (2013) Selection of time-domain features for fall detection based on supervised learning. In: Proceedings of the world congress on engineering and computer science, San Francisco, USA, 23–25 Oct 2013

261. Aguiar B, Rocha T, Silva J, Sousa I (2014) Accelerometer-based fall detection for smart-phones. In: IEEE International symposium medical measurements and applications, Lisbon, Portugal, 11–12 June 2014

262. Pannurat N, Thiemjarus S, Nantajeewarawat E (2014) Automatic fall monitoring: a review. Sensors 14(7):12900–12936

263. Cola G, Vecchio A, Avvenuti M (2014) Improving the performance of fall detection systems through walk recognition. J Amb Intel Hum Comp 5(6):843–855

264. Habib MA, Mohktar MS, Kamaruzzaman SB, Lim KS, Pin TM, Ibrahim F (2014) Smartphone-based solutions for fall detection and prevention: challenges and open issues. Sensors 14(4):7181–7208

265. Chen J, Kwong K, Chang D, Luk J, Bajcsy R (2005) Wearable sensors for reliable fall detection. In: Proceedings of the IEEE engineering in medicine and biology 27th annual conference, Shanghai, China, 1–4 Sept 2005

266. Chen K-H, Yang J-J, Jaw F-S (2016) Accelerometer-based fall detection using feature extraction and support vector machine algorithms. Instrum Sci Technol 44(4):333–342

267. Zhang T, Wang J, Xu L, Liu P (2006) Using wearable sensor and NMF algorithm to realize ambulatory fall detection. In: International conference on natural computation, Xi'an, China, 24–28 Sept 2006. Lecture Notes in Computer Science, vol 4222. Springer, Heidelberg, pp 488–491

268. Dinh C, Struck M (2009) A new real-time fall detection approach using fuzzy logic and a neural network. In: 6th International workshop on wearable, micro, and nano technologies for personalized health, Oslo, Norway, 24–26 Jun 2009

269. Li Q, Stankovic JA (2011) Grammar-based, posture-and context-cognitive detection for falls with different activity levels. In: Proceedings of the 2nd conference on wireless health, San Diego, USA, 10–13 Oct 2011

270. Gjoreski H, Lustrek M, Gams M (2011) Accelerometer placement for posture recognition and fall detection. In: 7th International conference on intelligent environments, Nottingham, UK, 25–28 July 2011

271. Noury N, Rumeau P, Bourke A, ÓLaighi G, Lundy J (2008) A proposal for the classification and evaluation of fall detectors. IRBM 29(6):340–349

272. Igual R, Medrano C, Plaza I (2013) Challenges, issues and trends in fall detection systems. Biomed End Online 12:66. https://doi.org/10.1186/1475-925X-12-66

273. Aziz O, Musngi M, Park EJ, Mori G, Robinovitch SN (2016) A comparison of accuracy of fall detection algorithms (threshold-based vs. machine learning) using waist-mounted tri-axial accelerometer signals from a comprehensive set of falls and non-fall trials. Med Biol Eng Comput 55(1):45–55

274. Bagalà F, Becker C, Cappello A, Chiari L, Aminian K, Hausdorff JM, Zijlstra W, Klenk J (2012) Evaluation of accelerometer-based fall detection algorithms on real-world falls. PLoS ONE 7(5):e37062

275. Deutsch M, Burgsteiner H (2016) A smartwatch-based assistance system for the elderly performing fall detection, unusual inactivity recognition and medication reminding. St Heal T 223:259–266

276. Ren L, Shi W (2016) Chameleon: personalised and adaptive fall detection of elderly people in home-based environments. Int J Sens Netw 20(3):163–176
277. Noury N (2002) A smart sensor for the remote follow up of activity and fall detection of the elderly. In: 2nd Annual international IEEE-EMBS special topic conference on microtechnologies in medicine and biology, Wisconsin, USA, 2–4 May 2002
278. Narayanan MR, Scalzi ME, Redmond SJ, Lord SR, Celler BG, Lovell NH (2008) A wearable triaxial accelerometry system for longitudinal assessment of falls risk. In: 30th Annual international conference of the IEEE engineering in medicine and biology society, Vancouver, Canada, 20–24 Aug 2008
279. Tiedemann A, Shimada H, Sherrington C, Murray S, Lord S (2008) The comparative ability of eight functional mobility tests for predicting falls in community-dwelling older people. Age Aging 37(4):430–435
280. Shany T, Redmond SJ, Narayanan MR, Lovell NH (2012) Sensors-based wearable systems for monitoring of human movement and falls. IEEE Sensors J 12(3):658–670
281. Podsiadlo D, Richardson S (1991) The timed "Up & Go": a test of basic functional mobility for frail elderly persons. J Am Geriatr Soc 39(2):142–148
282. Mathie MJ, Coster AC, Lovell NH, Celler BG, Lord SR, Tiedemann A (2004) A pilot study of long-term monitoring of human movements in the home using accelerometry. J Telemed Telecare 10(3):144–151
283. Shumway-Cook A, Brauer S, Woollacott M (2000) Predicting the probability for falls in community-dwelling older adults using the Timed Up & Go Test. Phys Ther 80(9):896–903
284. Zakaria NA, Kuwae Y, Tamura T, Minato K, Kanaya S (2015) Quantitative analysis of fall risk using TUG test. Comp Method Biomec 18(4):426–437
285. Lord SR, Menz HB, Tiedemann A (2003) A physiological profile approach to falls risk assessment and prevention. Phys Ther 83(3):237–252
286. Redmond SJ, Scalzi ME, Narayanan MR, Lord SR, Cerutti S, Lovell NH (2010) Automatic segmentation of triaxial accelerometry signals for falls risk estimation. In: Annual international conference of the IEEE engineering in medicine and biology, Buenos Aires, Argentina, 30 Aug–4 Sept 2010
287. Yusif S, Soar J, Hafeez-Baig A (2016) Older people, assistive technologies, and the barriers to adoption: A systematic review. Int J Med Inform
288. Kirchbuchner F, Grosse-Puppendahl T, Hastall MR, Distler M, Kuijper A (2015) Ambient intelligence from senior citizens' perspectives: understanding privacy concerns, technology acceptance, and expectations. In: De Ruyter B, Kameas A, Chatzimisios P, Mavrommati I (eds) Ambient intelligence. AmI 2015. Lecture Notes in Computer Science, vol 9425. Springer, Cham
289. Demiris G, Rantz MJ, Aud MA, Marek KD, Tyrer HW, Skubic M, Hussam AA (2004) Older adults' attitudes towards and perceptions of 'smart home' technologies: a pilot study. Med Inform Internet 29(2):87–94
290. Coughlin JF, D'Ambrosio LA, Reimer B, Pratt MR (2007) Older adult perceptions of smart home technologies: implications for research, policy & market innovations in healthcare. In: 29th Annual international conference of the IEEE engineering in medicine and biology society, Lyon, France, 22–26 Aug 2007
291. Jones S, Hara S, Augusto JC (2015) eFRIEND: an ethical framework for intelligent environments development. Ethics Inf Technol 17(1):11–25
292. Kötteritzsch A, Gerling K, Stein M (2016) Towards acceptance engineering in ICT for older adults. i-com 15(1):51–66
293. Chung J, Demiris G, Thompson HJ (2016) Ethical considerations regarding the use of smart home technologies for older adults: an integrative review. Annu Rev Nurs Res 34(1):155–181
294. Thilo FJ, Hürlimann B, Hahn S, Bilger S, Schols JM, Halfens RJ (2016) Involvement of older people in the development of fall detection systems: a scoping review. BMC geriatr 16:42. https://doi.org/10.1186/s12877-016-0216-3

295. Sprute D, Pörtner A, Weinitschke A, König M (2015) Smart Fall: accelerometer-based fall detection in a smart home environment. In: Geissbühler A, Demongeot J, Mokhtari M, Abdulrazak B, Aloulou H (eds) Inclusive smart cities and e-Health. ICOST 2015. Lecture Notes in Computer Science, vol 9102. Springer, Cham

296. van Vliet R, Hoang P, Lord S, Gandevia S, Delbaere K (2015) Multiple sclerosis severity and concern about falling: physical, cognitive and psychological mediating factors. NeuroRehabilitation 37(1):139–147

297. Van Doorn C, Gruber-Baldini AL, Zimmerman S, Richard Hebel J, Port CL, Baumgarten M, Quinn CC, Taler G, May C, Magaziner J (2003) Dementia as a risk factor for falls and fall injuries among nursing home residents. J Am Geriatr Soc 51(9):1213–1218

298. Allan LM, Ballard CG, Rowan EN, Kenny RA (2009) Incidence and prediction of falls in dementia: a prospective study in older people. PLoS ONE 4(5):e5521

299. Wildes TM, Depp B, Colditz G, Stark S (2016) Fall-risk prediction in older adults with cancer: an unmet need. Support Care Cancer 24(9):3681–3684

300. Mohile SG, Fan L, Reeve E, Jean-Pierre P, Mustian K, Peppone L, Janelsins M, Morrow G, Hall W, Dale W (2011) Association of cancer with geriatric syndromes in older Medicare beneficiaries. J Clin Oncol 29(11):1458–1564

301. Carr DB, Ott BR (2010) The older adult driver with cognitive impairment: "It's a very frustrating life". JAMA 303(16):1632–1641

302. Marottoli RA, Cooney LM, Wagner DR, Doucette J, Tinetti ME (1994) Predictors of automobile crashes and moving violations among elderly drivers. Ann Intern Med 121(11):842–846

303. Ohayon MM, Priest RG (1999) Night terrors, sleepwalking, and confusional arousals in the general population: their frequency and relationship to other sleep and mental disorders. J Clin Psychiatry 60(4):268–276

304. Bhattacharya SS (2002) Intelligent monitoring systems: smart room for patient's suffering from somnambulism. In: Annual international IEEE-EMBS special topic conference on microtechnologies in medicine and biology, Madison, USA, 2–4 May 2002

305. Kaur J, Molasaria N, Gupta N, Zhang S, Wang W (2015) Sleepstellar: a safety kit and digital storyteller for sleepwalkers. In: Proceedings of the 33rd annual ACM conference extended abstracts on human factors in computing systems, Seoul, South Korea, 18–23 Apr 2015

306. Singhal S, Jain P (2015) Wireless health monitoring system for sleepwalking patients. In: 39th National systems conference, Noida, India, 14–16 Dec 2015

307. De Lau LM, Breteler MM (2006) Epidemiology of Parkinson's disease. Lancet Neurol 5(6):525–535

308. Pringsheim T, Jette N, Frolkis A, Steeves TD (2014) The prevalence of Parkinson's disease: a systematic review and meta-analysis. Mov Disord 29(13):1583–1590

309. Kowal SL, Dall TM, Chakrabarti R, Storm MV, Jain A (2013) The current and projected economic burden of Parkinson's disease in the United States. Mov Disord 28(3):311–318

310. Arora S, Venkataraman V, Zhan A, Donohue S, Biglan K, Dorsey E, Little M (2015) Detecting and monitoring the symptoms of Parkinson's disease using smartphones: a pilot study. Parkinsonism Relat D 21(6):650–653

311. Zhan A, Little MA, Harris DA, Abiola SO, Dorsey E, Saria S, Terzis A (2016) High frequency remote monitoring of Parkinson's disease via smartphone: platform overview and medication response detection. https://arxiv.org/abs/1601.00960. Accessed Feb 2018

312. Contreras A, Grandas F (2012) Risk factors for freezing of gait in Parkinson's disease. J Neuroal Sci 320(1):66–71

313. Lamberti P, Armenise S, Castaldo V, de Mari M, Iliceto G, Tronci P, Serlenga L (1997) Freezing gait in Parkinson's disease. Eur Neurol 38(4):297–301

314. Achiron A, Ziv I, Goren M, Goldberg H, Zoldan Y, Sroka H, Melamed E (1993) Primary progressive freezing gait. Mov Disord 8(3):293–297

315. Bloem BR, Hausdorff JM, Visser JE, Giladi N (2004) Falls and freezing of gait in Parkinson's disease: a review of two interconnected, episodic phenomena. Mov Disord 19(8):871–884

316. Lieberman A, Deep A, Lockhart T, Frames C, Shafer S, McCauley M (2016) Why do patients with Parkinson disease fall? A single center experience. Neurology 86(16 Supplement):P4.330

317. Giladi N, Treves T, Simon E, Shabtai H, Orlov Y, Kandinov B, Paleacu D, Korczyn A (2001) Freezing of gait in patients with advanced Parkinson's disease. J Neural Transm 108(1):53–61

318. Perez-Lloret S, Negre-Pages L, Damier P, Delval A, Derkinderen P, Destée A, Meissner WG, Schelosky L, Tison F, Rascol O (2014) Prevalence, determinants, and effect on quality of life of freezing of gait in Parkinson disease. JAMA Neurol 71(7):884–890

319. Nonnekes J, Snijders AH, Nutt JG, Deuschl G, Giladi N, Bloem BR (2015) Freezing of gait: a practical approach to management. Lancet Neurol 14(7):768–778

320. Ando B, Siciliano P, Marletta V, Monteriù A (eds) (2015) Ambient assisted living: Italian Forum 2014. Springer International Publishing, Switzerland

321. Lim I, van Wegen E, de Goede C, Deutekom M, Nieuwboer A, Willems A, Jones D, Rochester L, Kwakkel G (2005) Effects of external rhythmical cueing on gait in patients with Parkinson's disease: a systematic review. Clin Rehabil 19(7):695–713

322. Hausdorff JM, Lowenthal J, Herman T, Gruendlinger L, Peretz C, Giladi N (2007) Rhythmic auditory stimulation modulates gait variability in Parkinson's disease. Eur J Neurosci 26(8):2369–2375

323. Keus SH, Munneke M, Nijkrake MJ, Kwakkel G, Bloem BR (2009) Phys Ther in Parkinson's disease: evolution and future challenges. Mov Disord 24(1):1–14

324. Jovanov E, Wang E, Verhagen L, Fredrickson M, Fratangelo R (2009) deFOG—A real time system for detection and unfreezing of gait of Parkinson's patients. In: Annual international conference of the IEEE engineering in medicine and biology society, Minneapolis, USA, 3–6 Sept 2009

325. Mazilu S, Hardegger M, Zhu Z, Roggen D, Tröster G, Plotnik M, Hausdorff JM (2012) Online detection of freezing of gait with smartphones and machine learning techniques. In: 6th International conference on pervasive computing technologies for healthcare (Pervasive Health) and Workshops, San Diego, USA, 21–24 May 2012

326. Maglogiannis I, Ioannou C, Tsanakas P (2016) Fall detection and activity identification using wearable and hand-held devices. Integr Comput-Aid E 23(2):161–172

327. Kim H, Lee HJ, Lee W, Kwon S, Kim SK, Jeon HS, Park H, Shin CW, Yi WJ, Jeon BS (2015) Unconstrained detection of freezing of Gait in Parkinson's disease patients using smartphone. In: 37th Annual international conference of the IEEE engineering in medicine and biology society, Milan, Italy, 25–29 Aug 2015

328. Tripoliti EE, Tzallas AT, Tsipouras MG, Rigas G, Bougia P, Leontiou M, Konitsiotis S, Chondrogiorgi M, Tsouli S, Fotiadis DI (2013) Automatic detection of freezing of gait events in patients with Parkinson's disease. Comput Methods Programs Biomed 110(1):12–26

329. Rezvanian S, Lockhart TE (2016) Towards real-time detection of freezing of gait using wavelet transform on wireless accelerometer data. Sensors 16:475. https://doi.org/10.3390/s16040475

330. Pepa L, Ciabattoni L, Verdini F, Capecci M, Ceravolo M (2014) Smartphone based Fuzzy Logic freezing of gait detection in Parkinson's Disease. In: IEEE/ASME 10th International Conference on mechatronic and embedded systems and applications (MESA), Senigallia, Italy, 10–12 Sept 2014

331. Pepa L, Capecci M, Verdini F, Ceravolo MG, Spalazzi L (2015) An architecture to manage motor disorders in Parkinson's disease. In: IEEE 2nd World forum on internet of things, Milan, Italy, 14–16 Dec 2015

332. Mazilu S, Blanke U, Dorfman M, Gazit E, Mirelman A, M Hausdorff J, Tröster G (2015) A Wearable assistant for gait training for parkinson's disease with freezing of gait in out-of-the-lab environments. ACM TIIS 5(1):5

333. Espay AJ, Bonato P, Nahab FB, Maetzler W, Dean JM, Klucken J, Eskofier BM, Merola A, Horak F, Lang AE (2016) Technology in Parkinson's disease: challenges and opportunities. Mov Disord 31(9):1272–1282

334. Pepa L, Verdini F, Capecci M, Maracci F, Ceravolo MG, Leo T (2015) Predicting freezing of gait in Parkinson's Disease with a smartphone: comparison between two algorithms. In: Andò B, Siciliano P, Marletta V, Monteriù A (eds) Ambient assisted living. Biosystems & biorobotics, vol 11. Springer, Cham

335. Bai L, Efstratiou C, Ang CS (2016) weSport: Utilising wrist-band sensing to detect player activities in basketball games. In: The 2nd IEEE international workshop on sensing systems and applications using wrist worn smart devices, Sydney, Australia, 14–18 Mar 2016
336. Schwab DJ, Haider CR, Felton CL, Daniel ES, Kantarci OH, Gilbert BK (2014) A measurement-quality body-worn physiological monitor for use in harsh environments. Am J Biomed Eng 4(4):88–100

Chapter 3
Ex Vivo Biosignatures

3.1 Introduction

Within the scope of biomedical science and sensors, an ex vivo biosignature can be defined as a description of a physiological phenomenon which extends from a colour cue up to signals and images recorded from the body using sensors that represent the physical and mental status of the human being (Fig. 3.1). The technical vision of mhealth for ex vivo biosignatures is to enhance the comfort of hosting the sensor system by reducing the number of contact sensors while boosting the number of attained psycho-physiological parameters, i.e. the significance of monitoring. This demands understanding the strategic approaches for classification of the ex vivo biosignatures based on their existence (permanent and induced), dynamic (quasi-static and dynamic) and origin (electric, magnetic, optic, thermal) [1]. In terms of existence, the emphasis is on permanent systems to eliminate the need for external triggers or excitation to acquire physiological data. However, if contactless data acquisition is not attainable, reducing the number of sensors, ideally to a single sensor, with wireless transmission to a smartphone is favoured. The dynamic nature of ex vivo biosignatures is another parameter of interest which determines the required time frame for monitoring; however, this parameter is case-specific. For example, the core body temperature is a quasi-static ex vivo biosignature which exhibits clinically low-value circadian rhythm in normal settings and thus daily readings suffice, whereas in the case of treatment for acute infection or post-op management, hourly-based monitoring might be required. This implies that a flexible, feedback loop-based mhealth platform is essential for applications in different short- and long-term settings. The physiological origin of ex vivo biosignatures conventionally governs the instrumentational approach for data acquisition; however, advances in biomedical sciences allows extracting various physiological data streams from a single ex vivo biosignature. For example, the heart rate (the number of contractions of the heart per minute; bpm) is typically extracted from the contact-mode cardio bioelectrical time signals, namely electrocardiogram (ECG). However, new state-of-art technologies

© The Author(s), under exclusive license to Springer Nature Switzerland AG 2019
G. Khalili Moghaddam and C. R. Lowe, *Health and Wellness Measurement Approaches for Mobile Healthcare*, SpringerBriefs in Computational Intelligence,
https://doi.org/10.1007/978-3-030-01557-2_3

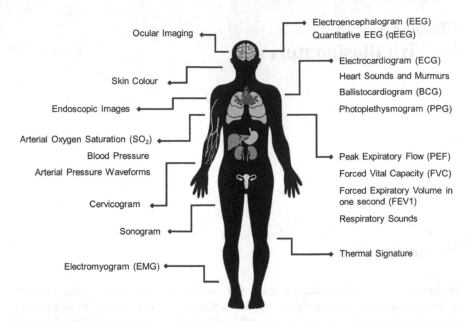

Fig. 3.1 Ex vivo biosignatures (*Note* This is not a comprehensive list)

enable contact-less heart rate monitoring using thermal- or colour-based biosignatures. Consequently, there is an emerging interest in the development of versatile sensor platforms for maximising the significance of monitoring are favoured in mhealth.

3.2 Sensor Technologies

The majority of technologies for monitoring ex vivo biosignatures rely on accessory sensors, wearables and smart biomedical devices that are linked to smartphones; one exception is the use of the embedded image sensor in smartphones. The remainder of this section explores existing sensor technologies in the realm of monitoring of ex vivo biosignatures (Fig. 3.2). It is noteworthy that these technologies exclude the platforms that still require further development to be appropriate for the mhealth vision, for example, radar-based sensors for biosignals [2].

3.2.1 Wearables

The capability and robustness of Internet-of-Things (IoT) in healthcare as well as data systems is increasing while the related development costs are falling. The sphere of embedded sensors in wearables has been extended to record heart rate based on

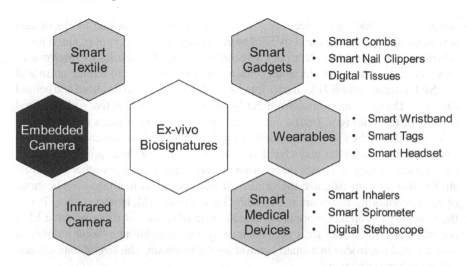

Fig. 3.2 Sensor technologies in mhealth for remote monitoring of ex vivo biosignatures

the photoplethysmography (PPG) methodology, where a combination of a dedicated optical emitter and a photodiode are used to measure the absorption of the light by sensing the cardiovascular blood volume pulse through transmitted light [3, 4].The reflectance time depends on the blood pulse rate which is determined by the heart rate that represents the time period between consecutive heart beats or QRS-complexes (the series of deflections in an electrocardiogram that represent electrical activity generated by ventricular depolarization prior to contraction of the ventricles). Accordingly, the photodiode receives a periodic signal for the duration of the measurement due to changes in the amount of reflected light during the cardiac cycle and hence, the heart rate is determined. While the availability of such wearable devices allows heart rate self-monitoring, there is still the challenge of user motivation. This issue has been considered by Han et al. [5] who synchronised the heart rate recording with a game on a smartphone. This technology is adaptable to video game controllers to monitoring the condition of players to enhance the game experience by enabling game scoring if the players keep calm [6]. Moreover, heart rate monitoring of gamers empowers game developers with a data-derived tool to analyse the behaviour of players and improve the game design using a more balanced concept [7]. Despite these pros, there are inherited drawback associated with the spot-based measurement [8].

Another category of wearables is smart head-sets/bands that record electroencephalogram (EEG) as an affordable, portable alternative to conventional electroencephalography [9–11]. This can enable measuring electric signals of the brain for both clinical EEG data acquisition and brain-computer interfaces with the aim of either communication or control wheelchair for those with severe motor impairment. Examples are NeuroSky® [12], Melon (acquired by DAQRI) [13], MUSE™ [14] and Emotive [15]. Although sound promising, reliability of EEG data collected using these portable solutions is a matter of concern. A conventional electroencephalography uses 20–200 "wet" electrodes (a conductive paste is applied to electrodes) across the scalp to record the activity of various brain regions. However, smart headsets utilise one to 14 "dry" electrodes to record brain signals; for instance, Melon uses two electrodes where the electrode configuration is optimised to reduce noise and MUSE has incorporated 7 electrodes into its headband across the forehead and behind each ear. The challenge stems from partly recording electrical activity of a limited regions of the brain (e.g. frontal cortex) and partly filtering artifacts due to muscle activity of the forehead and detachment of the device. To address this challenge, Emotive utilises 14 electrodes and a bandwidth filter (0.2–45 Hz) to acquire EEG which showed satisfactory outcomes for emotional studies. There are a few other individual studies that have investigated the validity of smart headsets in clinical applications of brain monitoring which are reviewed by Byrom et al. [16]. However, there is still the necessity to conduct more concise studies on reliability of these portable EEG recorders and optimising their performance by accommodating a larger number of miniaturised electrodes in a smart headset and/or increasing the size of datasets and relevant characterisations.

The other category of wearables that has attracted attention is for monitoring breathing rate and patterns. Breathing involves synchronised function of respiratory muscles especially the thoracic diaphragm. Accordingly, respiratory excursion can be monitored through the measurement of chest mobility using motion sensors in abdominal and thoracic wall positions [17, 18]. In this context, Spire [19] has developed a clip-on wearable (on belt or bra) that monitors the expansion and contraction of torso (abdomen) to derive the breathing pattern which can be classified into calm, focused or tense categories. This breath tracker costs US$99 including an app that offers notifications for breathing exercise when the user is tense. Although its performance sound promising, the design is not user-friendly and might create protrusion on the body.

3.2.2   Smart Textile

Another emerging IoT technology is smart clothing where body area network (BAN) systems are incorporated into clothing to monitor physiological signals using miniaturised electrodes with wireless transmission capability in real time. A wireless BAN can be integrated into the fabric of a garment by using conductive/electrostrictive fibres or silver nanowires. The nanowire system is "flexible and maintains the close contact" [20], and therefore enables more accurate biosignal monitoring than other technologies [21]. This platform, however, is not available in the market. Examples of existing garments incorporating interwoven textile electrodes for monitoring biosignals are HWM 200 Vital Jacket® [22], NTT [23], Wealthy [24], SmartVest [25], MagIC [26], Smart Shirt [27] and hWear™ [28]. The platforms differ in terms of usability (washable, stretchable), communication technology, gateway node (Smartphone, PDA), BAN topology (star, mesh and hybrid), power consumption and the number of sensor nodes. The systems also vary in terms of signal processing capabilities, with respect to removing muscle and motion artefacts and contact noise. However, being proprietary, their techniques are not open to critique. Jones and Martin [29] discuss hard- and software architecture of smart textiles in more detail.

A key issue in textile-based wearable system is the power consumption of the sensor nodes, which needs to be optimised specifically when continuous monitoring of a patient is required (i.e. epileptic seizures, heart rhythmic disturbances and sleep apnea). Traditionally the gateway node processes all serial data streams that are produced by sensor nodes. This implies that a major cause of power consumption at a sensor node is data transmission. Therefore, it is important to make a trade-off between local processing at sensor nodes and less communication to the gateway. Another factor affecting power consumption of sensor nodes is the topology of the network. In a WBAN (Wireless Body Area Network), nodes communicate with each other and thus it is essential to evaluate the efficiency of various network topologies for both powerful and weak nodes.

Most of the available smart textiles monitor ECG; however, there are challenges to assure it is entirely trustworthy for clinical interpretation. This implies that the recorded ECG signal should be of a reasonable quality and contains limited noise or artifactual components due to movements and muscle tremor during recording, or other external influences [30–32].

Smart clothing also has demonstrated significant growth and adoption monitoring electromyography (EMG) with applications as assistive and rehabilitation technologies as well as silent speech interface and input devices. EMG measures muscle action potential signal in response to a stimulation of nerve of the muscle and can be recorded using biopotential electrodes to assess the health of muscles and the nerve cells that control them (motor neurons), detect neuromuscular abnormalities and offer biofeedback for effective remote rehabilitation of stroke survivors. Finni et al. [33] embedded electrodes into clothing to monitor pattern of surface EMG (sEMG; using surface electrodes rather than needle electrodes) signals in real-time. Their study showed a good agreement (within 2SD) between textile and traditions electrodes in terms of the EMG signal amplitude and thus, demonstrated the feasibility of smart clothing for assessing the average rectified value of EMG. An example of commercially available smart shorts for measuring EMG activity is Mbody with six EMG channels [34]. Despite the promising research results of wearables for monitoring EMG, Düking et al. [35] consider smart shorts inaccurate for monitoring muscular activity due to drawbacks of skin electrodes including accurate positioning on the innervation zone [36, 37], configuration to cancel the effect of crosstalk and non-linearity of the signal-force relationship [36]. They suggested the use of pressure sensors into compression garments as a reliable approach to monitor muscle and limb activity [37]. However, a recent study on accuracy and reliability of EMG monitoring using smart shorts during three dynamic tasks (running, cycling and squatting) demonstrated comparable outcomes across smart shorts and conventional sEMG electrodes [38]. Nevertheless, there are still technical considerations to be taken into out in order to optimise the performance of smart shorts which are comprehensively reviewed by Hakonen et al. [39] including electrode configuration, electrode-to-electrode spacing, number of electrodes, electrodes placement, sampling rate of data acquisition and signal filtering and processing.

3.2.3   Smart Medical Devices

A transformative category of IoT in healthcare is smart medical devices which is projected to have a broad range impact on many sectors of healthcare. Examples of smart medical devices that are either commercialised or are in early commercialisation stages are investigated herein.

3.2.3.1   Smart Inhaler

Inhaler-based monitoring devices are an example of digitised healthcare [40–43]. Introducing the sensing compartment to inhalers began with an electronic monitoring accessory [44], which through the modernisation process has integrated into the inhaler. Kikidis et al. [45] present an extensive technical review on the evolution of smart inhalers between 1990 and 2015 and provides visions for the future development for unmet clinical needs. According to the report of Asthma UK, effectiveness studies are being conducted for large-scale investment of pharmaceutical companies in smart inhalers [46].

3.2.3.2   Smart Peak Flow Meter

Another category of smart devices for managing respiratory disorders are smartphone compatible measuring devices. Chamberlain et al. [47] used augmented reality to develop a machine vision-based app to capture the reading of conventional peak flow meters with a mean error of 5.7 L/min within 17.5 s. Although this app automatically creates an electronic record which addresses the burden of inconsistency and inaccuracy in manual asthma diaries, there is a trend towards smart peak flow meters and smart spirometers to measure, respectively, the rate and volume of air expelled from the lungs. The initial attempts to develop such devices were microcontroller-based with a flow meter detector and a Bluetooth transmitter or USB to record the data on a smartphone and subsequently, communicate with the healthcare professional [48–51]. To reduce the cost of the final product, the fixed orifice operating method, which only demands a pressure sensor, was considered by Bumatay et al. [52]. In this method the amplitude of the signal from a differential pressure sensor embedded in a tube was fed into a smartphone via the headphone jack to quantify the flow rate. However, the pressure differential was created using a small hole that may cause discomfort for the user due to resistance to airflow; this issue was addressed by Natarajan et al. [53] and the performance of the device was improved. There are also still-in-development [54, 55] and commercial [56, 57] devices, although the details on the principal functionality of the flow and volume sensors and/or respiratory measurements are not disclosed. The high price of existing commercial smart spirometers and peak flow meters has encouraged the emergence of innovative designs to combine various functionalities into one device. For example, Schneider [58] presented a novel smart device for personal asthma treatment that combines a spirometer and an inhaler with adjustable dosage, which also has incorporated ergonomic and semantic considerations. It should be noted that the performance of smart respiratory devices still needs to be approved by authorities to be certified as medical devices for evidence-based medical decisions.

3.2.3.3 Digital Stethoscope

The other example of smart devices is the digital stethoscope for enhancing auscultation through digitally recording the sounds of the heart and lungs. The basic characteristics of sound that applied to auscultations are amplitude and frequency. Body sounds occur at very low frequencies with only a fraction audible to the human ear and thus, their acquisition is challenging. Herein, body sounds refer to lung sounds (produced by vortical and turbulent flow within lung airways during inspiration and expiration of air) [59, 60] and heart sounds (produced by the flow of blood into and out of heart and by the movement of structures involved in this flow, such as heart valves) [61]. The acoustic performance of the stethoscope allows the identification and diagnosis of potential medical conditions. However, such diagnosis is subjective, implying that it depends on the technical properties of the stethoscope for optimised signal acquisition (amplification and noise reduction) and the skills of the healthcare professional to interoperate signs such as gallop rhythms [62]. The performance of stethoscopes has been enhanced by integrating digital compartments for sound amplification (up to $24\times$) [63], ambient noise reduction (up to 85%) [63] sound recording features and data transmission to smartphones for electronic documentation (Fig. 3.3). Elimination of ambient noise is a key factor in efficient phonocardiography and thus, the performance of various methods have been evaluated, including adaptive noise cancellation [64], adaptive line enhancement [65, 66], autoregressive modelling [67], merged adaptive line enhancement and band pass filtering [66], where the latter offers an enhancement of 14 dB in the range of 0–20 Hz. The digital stethoscopes are linked to apps for sound visualisation and signal/murmur processing, for example, using a heart and pulmonary sound reference library, as well as information sharing to seek peer advice or teaching. Gupta et al. [68] thoroughly describes the technical compartments of a typical digital stethoscope. It is noteworthy that assessing the signal quality is another critical task that demands incorporating an accurate pre-processing step to assure the signal is suitable for analysis by machine learning algorithms. This is particularly important in a situation that the phonocardiogram is acquired by untrained users. For instance, Das et al. [69, 70] analysed audio signals for classifying and discarding the noise phases from a continuously acquired signal with a sensitivity and specificity of 78.9 and 70.8%, respectively, which outperformed previous algorithms [71–73].

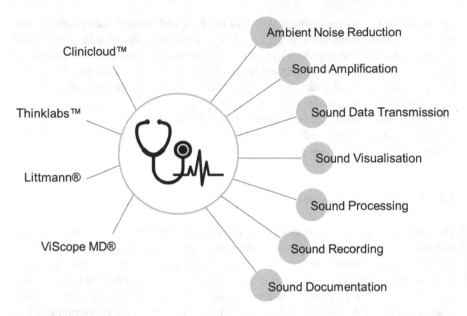

Fig. 3.3 Value-added features of digital stethoscopes and examples of commercially available brands

Digital stethoscopes are commercially available. For example, Clinicloud™ offers a pocket-size digital stethoscope without the bulky tubing that accommodates a 3.5 mm headphone jack for connection to a smartphone. A similar design is offered by Thinklabs™ with a Bluetooth transmitter for $599 USD [74]; however, professionals have reported suboptimal noise reduction in real-time auscultation. An alternative digital stethoscope that has been reported superior in performance is 3M™ Littmann® [63], which has a more conventional design with tubes. ViScope MD® is a digital stethoscope that has coupled an LCD screen to a conventional design of a stethoscope for digitised sound visualisation [75]. Sinharay et al. [76] used the principles of direct acoustic coupling to deploy an ultra-low cost accessory to convert a smartphone to a digital stethoscope; however, improving the noise reduction feature is required. Alternatively, 3D printing technology and off-the-shelf electronic components can be used to fabricate a low-cost digital stethoscope, where a 3D printed chest piece accommodates an electric microphone and the customised electronic board for sound amplification and filtering [77]. A dongle connects the chest piece to a smartphone through a headphone jack on which a graphical user interface displays phonocardiograms.

Alongside efforts for improving the design of digital stethoscopes, analysis approaches have been evolved to present an added-value to the interpretation of heart and breath sounds and murmurs. The research work on identifying heart diseases based on phonocardiography are largely classified into segmentation and unsegregated methods. The segmentation approach splits phonocardiograms into cardiac phases including two audible (S1, S2) and one rarely audible (S3) and not audible (S4) sounds [78–80]. The first sound (S1; systole) is due to closing of atrioventricular valves in the frequency range of 30–40 Hz; the second sound (S2; diastole) is due to closure of the semilunar valves in the frequency range of 50–70 Hz; the third sound (S3; ventricular gallop) is due to opening of the mitral valve after S2 in the frequency of ~30 Hz, and the fourth sound (S4) occurs at the end of S2 and before S1 at low frequency and intensity which makes it not audible [81]. The segmentation method either uses the electrocardiogram (ECG) as a reference [82–84] or an envelope-based algorithm, such as normalised average Shannon energy [85], Hilbert [modified] transforms [86–88] or homomorphic filtering [89], through three steps of extracting the envelope, detecting the peaks of the fundamental heart sounds and identifying the cardiac cycles with the peak conditioning. Once the heart sound is segmented, features of mechanical activity of the heart in one cardiac period are extracted and a classifier, hidden Markov models and neural networks, is exploited to identify abnormalities in the heart sound. Although the performance of the segmentation approach in identifying abnormalities is accurate, the presence of noise, for example, due to movement of the chest piece on the human body during data acquisition, poses a significant challenge to its efficiency. Analysing the entire unsegregated signal based on, for example, autocorrelation features and diffusion maps, can address this challenge but at the cost of reducing the relative accuracy [90, 91]. Although the performance of both approaches sound promising, there is concern regarding their validity because often variations across patient demography, devices and the position of the stethoscope on the human chest were not incorporated. Banerjee et al. [92] tackled this issue by evaluating the validity of a wide range of features in both time and frequency domains for various morphological and statistical settings and developed a robust dataset-agnostic classifier for phonocardiograms. However, this platform needs to be assessed on a more diverse dataset in the future.

3.2.3.4 Smart Sphygmomanometer

Other examples of remotely measurable clinical parameters using smart medical devices are arterial oxygen saturation and blood pressure. Examples of commercialised smart blood pressure monitoring devices (sphygmomanometers) are iHealth® (wrist-worn) [93] and Withings (arm-worn) [94] costing US$80 and US$130, respectively. A common source of error for automated measurement of arterial oxygen saturation and blood pressure is motion [95]. Relative motion between the probe and fingertip affects the optical path between LEDs and detector during monitoring the arterial oxygen saturation value, which can be addressed by incorporating an additional light source or accelerometer. Likewise, relative movement between the arm and the cuff of a remote blood pressure meter can cause a rustling sound which ultimately will lead to fallacious estimation of the blood pressure.

3.2.3.5 Smartphone-Based Ultrasound

Smartphone-based ultrasound has evolved rapidly in recent years as another example of smart medical devices. This technology is already cleared by the FDA for various clinical applications from abdominal to cardiac examinations. Smart ultrasounds provide comparable image resolutions to conventional ultrasound machines that cost over US$100K (US$10–20K a second-hand basic system) [96]. One of the commercially available smartphone-based ultrasound is MobiUS™ SP1 produced by Mobisante [97]. This pocket-size, lightweight smart ultrasound costs US$7495 and supports two types of transducers: 3.5–5.0 MHz suitable for abdominal, obstetrician-gynecologist and 7.5–12 MHz for vascular, small organs assessment. Philips offered a higher resolution system at a lower price with a cloud storage option [98]. The platform consists of the Lumify transducer which connects to the smartphone via USB connection. There are three types of Lumify probes suitable for various types of applications based on the central frequency; for example, Lumify S4-1 is for lung and abdomen. This system costs ~US$6000 which is also available through a monthly subscription model of $199 per month. The downside of Philips system is that there is no support for iOS. Butterfly iQ [99] set to further reduce the cost to enhance accessibility of smart ultrasounds to individual healthcare professionals in resource-limited settings by selling its device at under US$2000. While reducing price of the device is a strategic goal for most of product developers, Clarius [100] has focused on improving performance by increasing image resolution and incorporating colour doppler which wirelessly stream data to both iOS and Android devices. Clarius device has passed CE mark approval for examining all parts of the torso including the heart. However, this device costs US$6900–9900, depending on B&W (black and white) and colour options.

3.2.3.6 Digestible Electronics

The last example of medical devices is digestible electronics that have been developed to assess gastrointestinal conditions. One type of digestible electronics has embedded a miniaturised colour camera(s) and light source such as PillCam™ (11 mm × 26 mm) [101]. PillCam is a non-invasive alternative to endoscopy that assists with diagnosis of bleeding, malabsorption, chronic abdominal pain and chronic diarrhoea. Unlike endoscopy, PillCam is swollen like an ordinary capsule and thus it is painless and sedation free during the procedure. Once swollen with water, the disposable pill cam moves naturally through the digestive tract and takes two pictures every second for eight hours, transmitting image to a data recorder worn around the waist. During this time, the patient can walk about, without a hospital stay, and is allowed to resume most normal activities. Eight hours after ingesting the camera, patients return to the hospital to return the data recorder. Another type of digestible electronics that has common value-added features of PillCam consists of a sensor platform. A commercially available example is SmartPill™ [102] which measures gastrointestinal tract transit times to diagnose motility disorders such as gastroparesis and chronic constipation. SmartPill provides diagnostic data as it travels through the gastrointestinal tract including pressure, pH and temperature, gastric emptying time, colonic transit time and whole gut transit time.

3.2.3.7 Smartphone-Based Gadgets

Alongside the rapid growth of smart medical devices, there is an emerging trend in the development of smart gadgets to monitor wellbeing through health indices in everyday life. One example is the smart toothbrush to monitor state-of-use and dental hygiene, where the integrated motion, pressure and scrubbing sensors acquire the information about brushing patterns [103–112]. The data are transferred to a smartphone via Bluetooth to be visualised in real-time. Subsequently, the app advises the user to optimise the brushing style or educate children. The interactive brushing procedure can be subjected to further stimulation and fun by incorporating music or interactive video games. An improved tooth brushing style results in reducing the occurrences of cavities and gingivitis, which ultimately can lead to tooth decay or loss. Other possible metrics that a smart toothbrush can monitor are fluoride and discolouration. In the same category, smart tongue scrapers can be considered that allow screening salivary microbes [113]. Bacquet and Riemenschneider [113] suggest a wide range of smart gadgets and their potential advantages in monitoring wellbeing such as combs, nail clippers and tissues to monitor, dandruff density, quality of nails and mucus, respectively

3.2.4 Ambient Light Imaging

3.2.4.1 Ballistocardiography

Embedded image sensors in smartphones can be used to obtain clinically important features. In this way, cardiac beat can be monitored through ballistocardiography (BCG) by exploiting the subtle head motion due to Newtonian reactions induced by the influx of blood through the aorta with each cardiac cycle. The motion-based methods track selected feature points over time to monitor (Newtonian reactions and develop the feature trajectory that is later used for heart rate estimation.) [114–116]. Systematic reviews by Sikdar et al. [117] and Hassan et al. [118] describe the research developments in BCG. Accordingly, the state-of-the-art motion-based algorithm of Balakrishnan et al. [114] was enhanced by rectifying the noise due to non-rigid head motions, i.e. facial expressions [115] and lowering the computational power demand by reducing the number of feature points to one [116]. Motion-based algorithms outperform the colour-based ones because of their robustness to the on-plane head rotation and their operation range covers both grey-scale and colour videos. However, BCG is highly sensitive and vulnerable to voluntary head movements, and hence, urging the subject to avoid such movements might be challenging in real-world settings.

3.2.4.2 Imaging Photoplethysmography

An ambient light camera can be used for imaging photoplethysmography (iPPG), where changes in the skin colour in a time series caused by changes in the blood volume of vessels are used for measuring heart rate over a short-term monitoring period [119–124]. Jonathan and Leahy [125, 126] demonstrated the potential of iPPG from the video of a finger placed on the camera lens without additional force. These initial studies were followed by Kwon et al. [127] to evaluate the feasibility of iPPG on a video of a face, which have demonstrated that the camera of a smartphone has the potential to monitor heart rate in a medically reliable fashion (Fig. 3.4). The commercialisation potential of iPPG using smartphones is perceived by industrial stakeholders such as Philips [8]. iPPG is also applicable to a camera that is wirelessly connected a smartphone such as embedded cameras in unmanned aerial vehicles (drones) [128] which enable biomedical applications such as triage of disaster victims and the detection of security threats.

A general iPPG algorithm under controlled conditions initially detects the face of a still subject within the captured video frame followed by identifying the Region of Interest (ROI) which is a known location on the face. The descriptors of ROI are colour signals (red-green-blue; RGB) where each colour signal represents a different relative strength of the iPPG signal (pulse signal) [124]. The methods of extracting the pulse signal from the colour signals over multiple frames can be roughly categorised into (1) single channel green [124, 129, 130]; (2) combining two channels of red and green [131], and (3) blind source separation (independent/principal component analysis-based methods, which separate the temporal features to select the most periodic source as the pulse) [132–134]. Once the pulse signal is extracted, band-pass filtering is imposed to remove high- and low-frequency noises, as explained in a technical review by Rouast et al. [135]. Finally, the heart rate is estimated typically using either frequency analysis, such as fast Fourier transform [135], discrete cosine

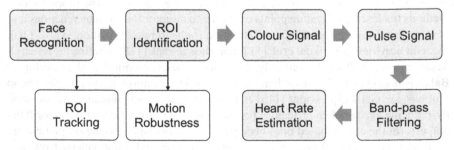

Fig. 3.4 A generic algorithm for imaging photoplethysmography (iPPG). The Region of Interest (ROI) is a predefined location on the face such as forehead

transform [116], Welch's method [129] or short-time Fourier transform [136] or peak detection, for example, cubic spline function [133, 137–139].

The promising outcome of iPPG under controlled conditions introduced the potential of a new course towards heart rate monitoring in mhealth: However, further performance enhancements are needed for the real-world applications. Herein, the focus is on pulse signal strength as well as motion- and illumination-robustness. Moreover, it is essential to evaluate the effect of technical characteristics across imaging devices on the performance of iPPG.

The contribution of pulse signal strength is important to maximising the signal-to-noise ratio. The amplitude of the pulse signal is mapped to the spatial average of pixels within the ROI, and thus, optimising the location of ROI on the face is essential. The location of the ROI varies among previous studies without a clear justification, including 60% of the full face [134], the forehead region [132] and an area below the eye line with a height and width of 20 and 55%, respectively [136]. Other studies [129, 130, 140–142] considered multiple ROIs to enhance the overall signal-to-noise ratio, which is a computationally expensive approach. Fallet et al. [143] performed a power spectral density analysis into 260 small facial ROIs to identify the locations that demonstrated more pronounced colour fluctuations induced by blood perfusion. Accordingly, the spatial distribution of heart rate information is more noticeable in the forehead region followed by the cheek region. The forehead is less vulnerable to voluntary movements compared to other areas of the face. Further studies are essential to validate these preliminary results across skins of different colour and the posture of the subject. It should be noted, however, that the feasibility of monitoring iPPG for various pigmentation densities (Asians, Africans and Caucasians) has been already demonstrated by Poh et al. [133, 134]. Another factor affecting the selection of ROI is the method of extracting the pulse signal from the colour signals. A comparison study by Sikdar et al. [117] has demonstrated that the forehead is favoured when nonlinear methods are used, whereas the full face provides a more promising performance for linear methods. The distance between the subject and the camera is another factor affecting the signal intensity which is typically considered <3 m. Long-range iPPG introduces unique challenges such as decreased light reflectance and smaller ROIs. A recent study by Blackford et al. [144] evaluated the possibility of increasing this distance to 25, 50 and 100 m where the mean absolute error for 1 min monitoring was respectively, 2, 4.1 and 10.9 bpm compared with the gold standard. The authors suggested improving the accuracy through enhanced lens power and subject illumination as well as optimising the bioprocessing methods for long-range measurements.

Once the location of the ROI is defined, it is necessary to track the ROI within consecutive video frames to ensure the efficient acquisition of colour signals which are invariant to head movements. This implies that ROI recognition and tracking algorithms are required to mitigate for subject movement. Different ROI tracking methods have been considered in previous studies, including manual selection [145, 146], Viola-Jones method [133, 134], Speeded-UP Robust Features method [147] and kernels method (CSK) [148]. An extensive review by Sun and Thakor [8] has identified the kernels method as superior in terms of tracking speed and reliability.

These tracking methods compensate the global motion artefact; however, the colour signals are still contaminated by motion artefacts. For example, generating pixel trajectories across the entire video may not be possible because some pixels may disappear due to occlusions such as rigid head movements, i.e. head tilting or rotation. Enhanced algorithms for extracting the pulse signal include: (1) CHROM (the pulse signal is a linear combination of chrominance signals assuming a standardised skin-colour to white-balance the camera) [149], (2) an adaptive colour difference operation between the green and red channels [147], (3) spatial redundancy [150], (4) PBV (a specific vector in a normalised red-green-blue (RGB)-space, namely $\vec{P}_{bv}$, defines the signature of blood volume change to extract pulse-induced colour changes from the averaged time-sequential RGB signals) [151] and (5) 2SR (spatial subspace rotation based on skin-pixel distribution in the image) [152]. While research on motion-robustness iPPG has been widely carried out, a recent study by Fan [153] demonstrated the feasibility of rectifying the errors due to intermittent appearance of ROI for 2–20 s using an adaptive hidden Markov model (a probabilistic algorithm) which led to implicit heart rate monitoring using the camera of a smartphone.

In addition to motion artefact attenuation, illumination-robustness is an indispensable task for iPPG in realistic conditions for two reasons. First, illumination variance can pose challenges to the performance of ROI tracking, particularly under extreme conditions, by creating spatial illumination variance, i.e. poorly illuminated regions, that affect the accuracy of the acquired colour signals. Arandjelović [154] offers a robust algorithm for face recognition under illumination changes, for example, sharp cast shadows, which requires only a single training image per individual. However, the efficiency of adapting such algorithms in iPPG under such extreme illumination changes are yet to be investigated. Second, the effect of illumination variance has a destructive impact on the performance of extracting the pulse signal from colour signals.

Previous attempts have demonstrated the feasibility of iPPG under constant lighting conditions, including ambient sunlight [155], fluorescent [147, 155], ambient sunlight-fluorescent combination [124, 156], quartz halogen [144] and poor ambient illumination [157]. One might argue in the case of using the built-in camera of smartphones, the white LED [158–162] can be considered as the dominant illuminant and thus, illumination changes might not be such a challenge. However, the crosstalk due to ambient artificial lights might be still a burden to monitor heart rate accurately using iPPG. For instance, the 100 Hz flicker frequency component from artificial lights in Europe (120 Hz in the US) [163] can be aliased down to frequencies which may be close to the heart rate. Tarassenko et al. [164] used a pole cancellation method to suppress strong aliased frequency components at around 4 Hz of the green-colour-signal caused by artificial light flicker, which allows iPPG to be followed under strong fluorescent lights. However, the pole cancellation method is not sufficiently robust to periodic variations due to its spectral analysis-based nature. Appearance-based models have shown the capability of compensating the effect of illumination changes on convex objects with a Lambertian reflectance function [165–167]; however, this approach demands a set of training images to form a convex cone in the image space under varying illumination conditions. Blanz et al. [168]

developed a morphable 3D model to encode shape and texture from a single facial image independent from imaging conditions (pose or illumination conditions), which is computationally demanding. Chen et al. [169] used the empirical mode decomposition method (Hilbert-Huang transform) to compensate the effect of ambient changes by decomposing reflectance from the green colour signal followed by decomposing intrinsic mode function. Based on a similar assumption that the mean green value of the ROI reflects the pulse signal and illumination changes, a normalised least mean square adaptive filtering method [129] and a multi-order curve fitting approach [170] were proposed to rectify the crosstalk due to temporal illumination changes. As an alternative, Cheng et al. [171] used a non-skin background as a reference to compensate the crosstalk based on the assumption that the ROI and background have similar illumination changes. The proposed illumination-robust algorithm was based on joint blind source separation and ensemble empirical mode decomposition, which rectified the crosstalk more efficiently than previous methods, and compared with the gold standard, resulted in the mean bias of 1.15 bpm with 95% limits and the correlation coefficient of 0.53.

In terms of technical characteristics, the impact of image quality, sampling rate and image resolution on the accuracy of heart rate estimation have been considered. The impact of image quality on the accuracy of iPPG was evaluated by assessing the capability of a high-performance CMOS camera and a low-cost webcam in measuring heart rate within the same experiments [145]. It was concluded that the heart rate measures of both setups were comparable with the gold standard, where the mean bias between these techniques was 0.33 bpm with 95% limits of agreement under various resting and exercise conditions. Sun et al. [145] also evaluated the effect of ambient light intensity due to weather conditions on the performance of both iPPG systems, which was not clinically noticeable. In the context of frame rate and image resolution, a comparative study on 9 synchronised cameras in a controlled head-motion experiments was carried out by Blackford and Estepp [172]. The sampling rates and image resolution were decreased, respectively, from 120 to 60 and 30 frames per second and 658×492 to 329×246 pixels (one quarter) using bilinear and zero-order down-sampling. A negligible difference in heart rate measurements was observed which allows the use of iPPG as an mhealth tool regardless of limited sampling rate to the frame rate of the camera (30 Hz), which is lower than gold standard electrocardiograms (125–1500 Hz). The matter of image resolution was further investigated by McDuff et al. [173] where the conventional video compression algorithms with a variable Constant Rate Factor was applied to the original captured video streams with the goal of reducing video bit-rates while preserving the iPPG data content. Although signal-to-noise was considerably decreased, the bit rate can be substantially lowered (10 Mb/s) without affecting the clinical data content (2.17 bpm estimation error), which would allow web streaming and bandwidth-limited applications.

An alternative approach to evaluate the effect of various enhancements and technical characteristics on the performance of iPPG is the use of computational models. Recently Wang et al. [174] developed a mathematical model for optimising the performance of robust algorithms for extracting the pulse signal through optical and physiological features of the model. The efficiency of this mathematical model was evaluated by introducing an algorithm for heart rate monitoring that outperformed the existing algorithms in terms of signal-to-noise ratio for various factors including skin tone (three skin types based on Fitzpatrick scale), motion (rotation and talking), luminance (single or a combination of fluorescent, red LED, green LED, blue LED, red-green LED, red-blue LED, green-blue LED) and recovery after a running exercise and fitness exercise (biking and stepping).

Although the potential of iPPG has been extensively discussed for heart rate monitoring, other research has extended its application to monitor respiration rate, oxygen saturation (SO_2) [119] and blood pressure with a single recording, which are thoroughly explained in systematic reviews [8, 175, 176]; of those, Daw et al. [176] focused on respiration rate monitoring in children.

3.2.4.3 Dermatology

The implication of ambient light imaging is also of utmost importance in dermatology. The importance of objective quantification of skin colour and its variations in dermatological practice and clinical research is widely recognised as colour cue can be used an indicator of skin diseases and condition [177, 178]; for example, total digital photography provides a means for early detection of melanoma [178]. A prerequisite for correct colour quantification and segmentation of skin lesions using digital imaging technology is controlling ambient lighting within the imaging laboratory [179, 180]. It is of particular importance for sequential colour measurements, where maintaining consistency during the assessment process provides meaningful comparison of clinical end points. Conventional platforms that integrate with a digital camera to control ambient lighting are ring-light/point through-the-lens flash systems and studio lighting systems [180], which have proved inadequate for the purpose of a low-cost and routine adjunct technology, implying that clinical digital photography is mainly used for monitoring high risk patients. To enhance its accessibility to clinicians being able to monitor a wide variety of patients, including young patients who are known to continue to develop new nevi, an image processing algorithm for estimating the ambient lighting from image data is desirable. Many colour constancy algorithms are passive and assume a linear model for the physical properties of the illuminants and objects which can lead to low estimation accuracy. Several methods have been suggested which use a standard reference colour card such as Munsell® Color MiniColorchecker to correct the image colour. This is a practical approach to estimate the ambient illuminant, although it needs an accessory calibration plate. A proposed algorithm by a research group at the University of Cambridge can be considered as an alternative accessory-free approach [181]. Once the colour of the captured image is corrected for ambient illumination, an automatic colour quantification is applied to classify the skin colour type based on the Fitzpatrick scale. This step is followed by automatic skin lesion segmenting and counting, after optimisation of the threshold of the feature vector. The combination of pre-processing and segmentation algorithms, enhance the efficacy of lesion border detection and thus improves the performance of automatic lesion segmentation methods, particularly in difficult-to-assess melanoma categories with complex patterns and variegated appearance, and therefore reduces the need for biopsy and expensive clinical imaging techniques.

3.2.4.4   Ophthalmology

Another application of ambient imaging is in eye care where the built-in camera of smartphones is used for clinical evaluation of the vision based on a standalone mode or using accessories such as magnifying lenses. This approach is valuable for acquiring ocular images with clinically-acceptable quality to diagnose diseases and monitor progression to prevent treatable causes of blindness in various settings, particularly in areas lacking reliable transportation or access to healthcare facilities. Garg [182] used a plastic housing encompassing a prism to align the path of the flash with the field of view of the camera and developed a direct ophthalmoscope to capture images of optic disks. The image acquisition feature can be combined with the processing power of smartphones to develop a platform for automated determination of the cup-to-disc ratio in order to objectively assess the progression of glaucoma (a blinding condition characterised by a loss of the optic nerve neuroretinal rim). Giardini et al. [183] demonstrated the potential of smartphone-based direct ophthalmoscopy in glaucomatous disk grading. EyeNetra has developed a pinhole optic including a film and a lens that clips onto the top of a high-resolution smartphone (e.g. Sony Xperia U) for measurement of refractive errors by exploiting alignment as an indicator of de-focus [184, 185]. An alternative vision screening approach used a Shack-Hartmann wavefront aberrometer extension to assess the refractive error [186]. The working range of these platforms is limited (e.g. −12.5 to +5.5 D for EyeNetra) and further developments are required. Another smartphone-based platform in ophthalmology is a miniaturised pupilometer (Smart Ophthalmics©) that allows pupillary light reflex and dark reaction by recording pupillary behaviour of both eyes at 120 Hz [187, 188]. The server-based analysis of Smart Ophthalmics© provides information such as dilation times, constriction and pupillary latency where the measurement of pupillary reactivity can also be used to assess patients with acute brain lesions [189]. The embedded camera in smartphones also appears promising for retinal imaging to examine fundus. Lord et al. [190] explored the possibility of fundus imaging through a slit-lamp ocular with a 78 D lens and a 20 D indirect lens. The latter required directing a pen touch light that may not appeal to ophthalmologists. This issue of smartphone-based fundoscopy was addressed by Bastawrous [191] where fundus images were captured using the inbuilt flash of the smartphone as a coaxial light source though a condensing lens (20 or 28 D). The photobiological safety of the iPhone 4 light source for indirect fundoscopy was investigated by Kim et al. [192] who demonstrated that the light levels are 150 times below thermal hazard limit and 240 times below the photochemical hazard limit by the International Organisation for Standardisation (ISO 15004-2.2). Haddock et al. [193] integrated the proposed platform by Bastawrous [191] with an app to control the focus, exposure and light intensity during video recording using an iPhone 4 and 5 (5 and 8 MP) to stabilise the image and reduce glare, which ultimately led to capturing high resolution fundus images. These findings were confirmed by Jalil et al. [194] who compared the performance of iPhone 4s and 5s with the RetCam II fundus imaging platform. The feasibility of adapting this platform to a more cost-effective smartphone (e.g. Tecno phantom A+; 8 MP) was clinically evaluated in Sub-Sahara Africa [195]. In a recent study, the possibility of fundoscopy using a smartphone model Blackberry Z-10 (8 MP camera) was assessed in both adults and children including branch retinal vein occlusion with fibrovascular proliferation, chorioretinal scarring from laser photo-coagulation, presumed ocular toxoplasmosis, diabetic retinopathy, retinoblastoma, and ocular albinism with fundus hypopigmentation [196].

3.2.4.5   Cervicography

The rear camera of smartphones can be integrated into an extension for cost-effective cervical screening by photographically reproducing colposcopy, which is a recom-mended strategic screening method by WHO [197]. Previous studies have demon-strated the feasibility of a range of camera-enabled mobile phones from 5 to 16 MP imaging resolutions in cervicography [198–201]. Parham et al. [200] reported chal-lenges in capturing appropriate images such as blurred images due to inadequate focus, orange colour casting due to low battery and shadows due to inadequate light-ing; trouble-shooting approaches were effectively implemented. One may argue the quality of images may affect the decision-making processes [111]. Four specialists rated a dataset of 258 images, and overall, 4.5, 42.6 and 52.9% were graded as inad-equate for interpretation, clinically acceptable and excellent, respectively [199]. A recent study by Gallay et al. [201] evaluated the quality of images (sharpness, focus and zoom) acquired by a 16 MP smartphone for making clinical decisions; 93.3% of cases were considered as adequate quality with an interobserver agreement of 0.45, which corresponds to a moderate agreement on the common scale of kappa values.

3.2.5   Thermal IR Imaging

The thermal infrared (IR) technology for the monitoring of psychophysiological activities is unlike that for physical activity that demands costly infrastructure to capture images of the entire body movements. For example, a lightweight thermal IR camera as a smartphone accessory (e.g. FLIR ONE® PRO; 36.5 g; 68 × 34 × 14 mm [202]) is sufficient to capture facial biothermal signals. Accordingly, thermal IR facial imaging is the technology that fulfils mhealth requirements in terms of acceptable price and robustness and yet is stable, easily adaptable and expandable. This technology demonstrates a contact-free system that is independent of changes in illumination, skin colour, facial extrinsic factors and environmental noises such as smoke or mist while, at the same time, being applicable to both day and night time applications. An IR camera may be used to collect facial biothermal signals and send them to a built-in and/or smartphone-based processor. Real-time processing of thermal imaging data in combination with data classification using artificial intelligence can potentially provide computational physiological data. IR radiation is energy radiated by all materials which are above 0 degrees Kelvin (−273 °C). According to the Stefan and Boltzmann equation, the intensity of the emittance through all wavelengths is a function of the temperature:

$$W = \epsilon.\sigma.T^4 \tag{3.1}$$

where W is radiant emittance (W/cm^2), ϵ is emissivity, σ is Stefan-Boltzmann constant (5.6705 × 10^{-12} W/cm^{2}K^4) and T is temperature in Kelvin. For human skin, ϵ is estimated at 0.985–0.990, which is higher than most other materials and which facilitates differentiating human skin from the background in IR images. It is known that the human skin emissivity varies as a function of wavelength and the maximum occurs at 10.6 μm. Accordingly, to maximise the precision of emission measurement, it is desirable to use a forward-looking infrared (FLIR) camera which operates within the long-wavelength infrared range (LWIR; 8–14 μm) [203]. Imaging in the LWIR band is also advantageous in terms of potential biohazards. Other IR bands require a light source which may irritate the target skin, whereas the LWIR imaging is passive in nature. The FLIR camera converts the IR energy into an electrical signal by the imaging sensor (microbolometer) in the camera and displays it on a monitor as a colour or monochrome thermal image. Recent advances in the technology for thermal IR imaging have provided commercially available high spatial/temporal resolution (640×480 pixels/~30 Hz) and high thermal sensitivity (~4 mK at 30 °C in the spectral range of 7.5–13 μm) devices. Such devices enable real-time contactless biothermal imaging for various applications in mhealth.

Monitoring facial biothermal signals allows extracting a wide range vital signs including localised blood flow, cardiac pulse and breath rate [204]. The dissemination of the pressure wave due to the ventricular systole through the arterial tree generates the arterial pulse which is correlated to the variations on the thermal signal of a superficial vessel. Accordingly, the frequency of thermal modulation representing pulse can be obtained by applying Fast Fourier Transform to points of interest along the vessel followed by an adaptive estimation function on the average Fast Fourier Transform [205]. Two major challenges in biothermal signal processing are low signal-to-noise ratio in low quality thermal IR cameras and subject tracking for accurate temporal recording. These challenges have been addressed by introducing further processing steps for noise reduction and automatic tracking of the vessel of interest, which improved the accuracy of performance from 88.6% to 95.3% [206–209]. In spite of the relatively high accuracy, the number of used video frames for analysis was 2000–3000 at 30 fps. Moreover, these studies were aimed at extracting the dominant heart rate frequency and hence, further research was carried out by Chekmenev et al. [210] to decouple the actual heart rate waveform using a wavelet-based approach, which achieved an average accuracy of 86.3%. However, the number of subjects was limited (<10), the impact of head movements was not considered and the selection of the vessel of interest was manual. Using more robust filtering and wavelet analyses on 30 subjects, Gault et al. [211] improved the selection of the vessel of interest from manual to a semi-automatic mode with an average accuracy of 93% on one arterial selection per subject. Afterwards, a fully automated approach to extract the arterial pulse waveforms using 512 frames with an accuracy of 85% was introduced by Gault and Farag [212]. Regardless of these improvements, further work is required to compensate various parameters such as spontaneous movements and thermal distortions including sweating and airflow.

IR thermography can also be used for measuring breathing rate and pattern. Breathing has a spatiotemporal thermal signature consisting of inspiration and expiration cycles in the proximity of the nostrils which is typically distinguishable from the background temperature of indoor environments. The feasibility of this approach was first evaluated by Murthy and Pavlidis [213] who introduced a statistical-based approach to quantify the breathing rate from biothermal signals with an average accuracy of 96.4%. However, this accuracy was obtained for experiments under strictly controlled conditions which imposed various practical limitations. For example, the proposed algorithm did not track the head position or the source of airflow (nasal or mandible) and thus, signal acquisition would be interrupted if the nostrils were not within the field of view of the camera. Fei and Pavlidis [214] integrated head tracking into a wavelet-based algorithm which ultimately enhanced the monitoring performance equivalent to that of a contact thermistor; however, they only used the biothermal signals around the nostrils. Later the head tracking feature was integrated into both nasal and mandible airflows because the latter is common in adults [215]. Despite the progress in quantification of breathing rates in resting conditions for healthy subjects, the performance in real-world settings might be challenging because physical activity or breathing disorders affect the breathing rate/waveforms. Various studies have been conducted to investigate the accuracy of breathing-related biothermal monitoring. Pereira et al. [216] compared the performance of breathing rate monitoring using biothermal signals with the gold contact standard method in three experimental groups including normal breathing with and without head movements and a sequence of specific breathing patterns. The results show that monitoring of biothermal signals allows accurate estimation of breathing rate under such conditions where the mean correlation with the gold standard was >0.94. This study was conducted on healthy subjects who mimicked various breathing patterns; however, the findings were confirmed by a study on adult patients who had diagnosed of obstructive sleep apnea by the gold standard method [217]. The application of monitoring biothermal signals was also extended for other clinically important respiratory metrics. Lewis et al. [218] demonstrated the possibility of estimating the relative tidal volume. These studies evaluated the performance of monitoring breathing rates and patterns in controlled temperature environments such as home and clinics. Although it is expected the adaptive statistical methods tolerate the rapid temperature changes that are more likely to happen in outdoor monitoring, the practical efficiency still should to be established.

3.3 Clinical Implications

A wide range of health symptoms and psychological states can be evaluated by extracting the required features from ex vivo biosignatures. For example, heart rate variability (HRV) which is the variation of time in milliseconds between two heartbeats can be used as a biomarker to rate the general health index, e.g. physiological stress results in an increase in HRV, whereas diabetes and obesity reduce HRV [219]. This index is found to predict mortality, morbidity and other health outcomes [220], while it is associated with physical and mental health indicators such as functional ability, depression as well as social risk factors such as socioeconomic status [221, 222]. In this section, the impact of advances in sensor technologies and cloud computing on tackling the burden of various categories of diseases and disorders is discussed.

3.3.1 Vascular Diseases

Vascular diseases are a leading cause of morbidity and premature mortality in developed countries [223, 224]. The deteriorated vascular functions would have generally become irreversible after being diagnosed and this necessitates the development of an assistive tool to support healthcare professionals with prognostic and diagnostic information. The two principal clinical markers of cardiovascular diseases (CVDs) are heart rate variability and breathing rate, both of which can be monitored though mhealth solutions (Fig. 3.5a, b). CVDs is a group of conditions that affect heart and blood vessels including angina and myocardial infraction, heart failure, arrhythmia and heart valve problems. A short-term (5 min) measure of HRV enables the real-time monitoring of cardiovascular function and therefore, enables detection of CVDs at an earlier stage before the occurrence of common clinical symptoms and organic lesions [225, 226]. Low HRV is associated with a 32–45% increased risk of a first cardiovascular event in populations without known CVDs [227]. The HRV monitoring also is also used in the fields of sport and sports science; for example, it is of the utmost importance in scuba diving where CVDs account for a quarter of diving fatalities [228–230]. Likewise, integrating the HRV monitoring system is beneficial to reduce the rate of fatal motor vehicle accidents. A road traffic analysis report showed that, in 2008–2009, sudden driver illness contributed to at least 8% of fatal motor vehicle accidents and 11% of driver deaths were attributable to a disease, mainly CVD [231, 232]. Another critical clinical metric for early diagnosis of CVDs is the breathing rate. A respiratory rate of 27 breaths/min has been reported as the most important predictor of cardiac arrest [233] and thus the fusion of heart rate and breathing rate measurements is likely to be a better means to diagnose CVDs early.

The clinical implications of mhealth for vascular events can also be mapped to the cloud computing strategic point (Fig. 3.5c). Biosignals as the raw data that are obtained from conventional biomedical instruments, such as Holter, contain valu-

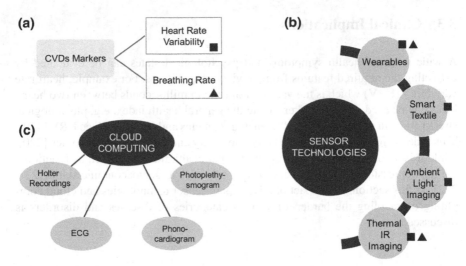

Fig. 3.5 a Clinical markers of cardiovascular diseases (CVDs), **b** sensor platforms of the mhealth strategy for remote monitoring of CVDs markers, heart rate variability and breathing rate, **c** the implicaton of cloud computing on enhancing prognosis and diagnosis of CVDs

able clinical and subclinical information. However, the subclinical data cannot be directly extracted, and thus, advanced mathematical methods and algorithms are required. The possibility of automatic prediction of cardio- and cerebro-vascular incidents using data mining algorithms, such as tree-based classifiers, support vector machines and artificial neural networks has been investigated. These methods are applicable to both echographic parameters and the HRV of Holter recordings; however, the latter is favoured as a risk stratification tool to identify high-risk hypertensive patients where sensitivity and specificity rates of 71.4 and 87.8%, respectively, were obtained [234]. Similarly, the time series entropy estimation methods including, but not limited to, fuzzy entropy (FuzzyEn) and sample entropy (SampEn), have been used to analyse ECG [235]. Despite their impressive implementation, there have been attempts to enhance further the stability and robustness of these entropy-based methods against noise while extending the range of measurable metrics to introduce additional clinical applications. Yentes et al. [236] compared the efficiency of approximate entropy and SampEn for short data sets and apparently, SampEn is more appropriate because of its lower sensitivity to changes in data length. Ji et al. [237] used a refined FuzzyEn method to assess changes of diastolic period variability based on short-term (5 min) recordings. This allows distinguishing patients with CVD from the healthy individuals, which was not achievable using conventional FuzzyEn and SampEn.

mHealth solutions are likewise beneficial to junior doctors for identifying abnormal heart sounds during phonocardiography. Newly graduated medical professionals are capable of identifying 15–20% of abnormal heart sounds [68], whereas phonocardiography is essential in regular check-ups. Digital stethoscopes empower junior

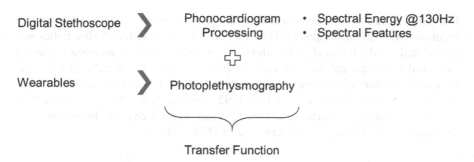

Fig. 3.6 mHealth solutions including sensor technologies and cloud computing, facilitate the identification of coronary artery disease (CAD) for junior doctors

professionals with a software package to analyse the audio signals for abnormalities such as coronary artery disease (CAD) which is a subtype of CVDs and mainly affects the coronary arteries which perfuse the heart muscle. CAD is due to building of plaque on the walls of coronary arteries which causes a heart attack due to the restricted blood flow. CAD is largely associated with proliferation of sedentary life styles, ageing and unhealthy diets and has led worldwide to more than one million deaths annually. CAD is clinically diagnosed using echocardiography, angiography and exercise stress testing, which are expensive and demand substantial healthcare infrastructures. Coarse clinical markers for the non-invasive diagnosis of CAD are based on prolonged HRV monitoring and phonocardiography [238]. The latter is attainable using a digital stethoscope, where biosignal processors detect abnormalities in the sound of opening and closing of heart valves (Fig. 3.6). For example, the spectral energy of CAD patients is higher than in normal individuals at a frequency of 130 Hz [78]. Banerjee et al. [239] exploited support vector machines to differentiate CAD patients and healthy subjects from spectral features of phonocardiograms with an accuracy of 80%. Moreover, they showed the possibility of identifying CAD using a simple transfer function, where the photoplethysmography (PPG) and phonocardiogram are acquired simultaneously at the same sampling rates. This approach is based on the closed-loop characteristics of the human body. Accordingly, phonocardiograms as the input to the cardiovascular system and PPG as the output are correlated through a transfer function which is different in CAD patients compared to healthy individuals. Thus, an adaptive filter with temporal adjustable features can be considered as a CAD marker. However, further research on noise reduction to boost the overall confidence score of phonocardiogram-PPG fusion is necessary.

Besides vascular diseases, the proposed contactless heart rate monitoring services of mhealth are valuable in the neonatal intensive care unit, particularly for very preterm infants whose fragile skin is prone to injuries and infections using contact methods such as electrocardiography and pulse oximetry. The feasibility of heart rate monitoring using an ambient camera has been evaluated at a distance of 1 m from infants for time periods of up to 5 min [139] and 7 h [240]. The outcomes appear promising; however, optimising the algorithm to address the challenge of low ambient lighting (3–6 lx in a covered incubator and 60–120 lx in an uncovered incubator with dimmed lights [241]) demand further development. This matter was considered by McDuff et al. [139] who used an advanced five-band ambient camera to record two extra colour features of cyan and orange and thereby increase the frequency resolution of recorded images. Their results are more aligned to the FDA guidelines where a correlation of over 0.92 with the gold standard contact PPG method was obtained. A more promising alternative approach is the thermal imaging for heart rate monitoring on pre-term infants [164, 241].

3.3.2   Respiratory Disorders

The existing clinical approaches for diagnosis and monitoring respiratory disorders are contact modalities (pneumotachometer, strain gauge and photoplethysmography) which introduce practical challenges such as discomfort and misalignment of sensors particularly during monitoring sleep disorders [216, 242–246]. Biothermal monitoring offers not only a contactless approach to address these challenges but also it can potentially be integrated into the mhealth ecosystem given the recent advances in the development of IR thermal accessories for smartphones. This mhealth service enables remote diagnosis of respiratory dysfunction based on abnormal breathing rates or atypical waveforms (Fig. 3.7). For example, Pereira et al. [216] verified the capability of this approach for identifying the simulated breathing patterns of eupnea (normal breathing) [247], tachypnea (high breathing rate) [248], apnea (low breathing rate) [249], Kussmaul breathing (regular rhythm but increased rate and depth) [249] and Cheyne-Stokes respiration (gradual increase followed by gradual decrease in depth and rate and a period of apnea) [249]. Moreover, unlike commercially available thermistors, biothermal monitoring allows quantification of relative tidal volume [218] and thereby enables differentiating between restrictive and obstructive pulmonary diseases. These respiration measures are of critical importance in both clinical and psychophysiological evaluations. For example, biothermal monitoring meets the criteria for an effective, low-cost, home-based apnea diagnostic, which has a prevalence of 20–50% in adults [250–252]. Early and effective diagnosis of apnea is of vital importance because of its association with various diseases including hypertension, coronary artery disease, heart rhythm disorders, pulmonary hypertension and stroke [253, 254]. The use of gold-standard polysomnography requires access to sleep laboratories, expensive equipment and trained technicians. Moreover, the deficiency of this diagnostic method is more pronounced in specialised groups with impaired mobility and neurocognitive function, such as early post-stroke patients [255], while early post-stroke patients have a higher prevalence of apnea compared to the general population (obstructive apnea: 3–7% vs. 30–70% [256] and central apnea: 1% vs. 6–26% [257, 258]). Although these limitations can potentially be addressed by lightweight monitoring devices such as BresoDx® [255], acoustic face frame [259], and single-channel nasal pressure [260], they can disturb sleep quality. Moreover, they are designed for short-term monitoring, whereas long-term, real-time screening is

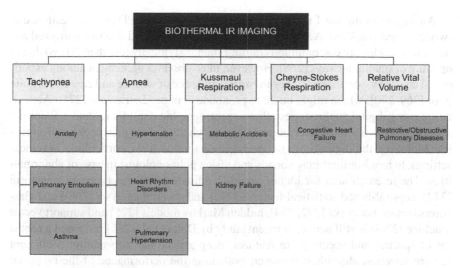

Fig. 3.7 Application of biothermal IR imaging in identifying various respiratory disorders and examples of their underlying causes

required, particularly in infants because the central apnea is one of the major causes of Sudden Infant Death Syndrome [261]. Hence, there is an increasing demand for the development of an unobtrusive, contactless and user-friendly approach for effective home-based diagnosis with long-term monitoring adaptability. Alkhin et al. [262] suggested bioradiolocation contactless screening of apnea, but it demands extensive instrumentation. Biothermal breathing rate monitoring meets the ideal requirements which would enhance effective diagnosis of apnea even in specialised groups and which eventually increases the health-related quality of life of patients, regardless of severity [263]. Additionally, it is expected that the implementation of this biothermal-based mhealth service allows optimisation of assignment to the in-lab assessment and, ultimately, reduces the wait times for the in-lab assessment, at least, from 152 days in average to 92 days [264]. An economic study on the cost of diagnosis and management of obstructive apnea in a high-risk population at home using a conventional method demonstrated a $264 per patient cost saving from the payer perspective, but a negative operating margin for providers [265]. However, fewer costs from both perspective are expected using the proposed biothermal-based mhealth service with a feedback loop because it meets the ideal criteria that enhances adherence and health outcomes. Moreover, the expected higher adoption rate of this 'ideal' apnea diagnostic approach with a cloud-based health record can facilitate studying the national and international trends and factors (e.g. obesity), which encourages policy makers to consider evidence-based management strategies [266]. Also, this mhealth service has the potential to address the under diagnosis of apnea, and thus, suppress the associated complications and burden [267].

An important marker for obstructive airway disease (COPD) is the breath sound (wheezes and crackles). A wheeze is a continuous lung sound due to a narrowed airway and crackles are discontinuous rattling sounds (typically less than 20 ms) due to opening of smaller airways [268]. However, inter-observer agreement among experienced chest physical therapists regarding the presence of wheeze and crackles is quite poor [269, 270], which might be more pronounced in paediatric care [271]. Auscultation using digital stethoscopes allows spectrographic analysis to detect abnormal sounds objectively and describe audiological characterises of wheeze and crackles. Moreover, the digital stethoscope empowers individuals, particularly in remote settings, to monitor their lung sounds and visit a pulmonologist in case of abnormalities. The research area for identifying discriminative features (wavelet transform [272], cepstral-based statistical features [273] and spectral analysis [268]) and classifiers (neural networks [272, 274], hidden Markov models [275] and support vector machine [276]) is still active. A recent study by Datta et al. [276] proposed a robust set of spectral and spectrogram features using a maximal information coefficient feature selection algorithm; however, evaluating the performance of the proposed algorithm on a more diverse dataset and the feasibility of classifying abnormalities requires further research. The feasibility of digital stethoscope-based mhealth services also has been investigated in children across a variety of ages (4.6–17.1 years) using standard and two models of digital stethoscopes (i.e. Littman 3200 and Clinicloud) [277]. Concordance between standard auscultation and each Littman and Clinicloud for wheeze detection was 75 and 80%, respectively, while concordance of 100% was obtained for crackle detection for both digital stethoscopes, which is classified as almost perfect based on kappa interpretation. The moderate agreement between conventional and digital stethoscopes stems from the intrinsically superior performance of digital ones.

3.3.3 Asthma

The benefits of continuous monitoring of breathing rate and patterns using wearables and thermal IR imaging for enhancing diagnosis and monitoring respiratory disorders discussed in the previous section. However, mhealth solutions including smart respiratory devices and associated apps, can also contribute towards the management of respiratory disorders, particularly asthma (Fig. 3.8). Asthma is costly; for example, £108M is spent every year in the UK on consultations for asthma [46]. The global number of people with asthma is currently 235M [278] and it is expected to reach 400M by 2025 [279], which will lead to an increase in the associated socioeconomic burdens and thus healthcare providers are considering strategies to supress the underlying causes of sub optimised asthma self-monitoring. Poor asthma control is associated with a lack of education or awareness; 25% of patients are unaware of the symptoms of asthma and 19% are not able to identify worsening signs [58]. Educational apps can encourage awareness of symptoms and disseminate information about the right usage of medication. However, the asthma condition is not only about symptoms, i.e. asthma attacks, but also demands a combination of symptom awareness and quantified measures. Accordingly, one of the main elements in asthma control is documentation, such as peak flow diaries, which allow early evaluation of symptoms and provide feedback about the level of symptom control. Moreover, among asthmatics, about 50% do not take their medication as prescribed [46] and two thirds of them do not attend their asthma review [280]. Such lack of adherence causes two thirds of asthma-related deaths which are preventable [281]. Accordingly, one strategy to contain the asthma burden is enhancing engagement with a management plan. Pinnock et al. [282] investigated the impact of mhealth on asthma self-monitoring. Accordingly, mhealth can boost confidence and understanding of asthma management in the early phase while enabling cloud-based records of peak flow readings that can be shared with the consultant to arrange appointments when necessary. Although the reading of peak flow can be communicated manually through apps, the recent advances in the field of respiratory devices allows integrating digital features with smartphone compatibility that enables uploading data to the cloud via the smartphone. Moreover, the strategy of implementation of smart technologies, such as smart inhalers, after clinical approval have the potential to enhance asthma outcomes by offering personalised asthma management plans based on objective monitoring of medication use [283–285]. For instance, Heaney and McGarvey [286] showed that optimising asthma self-monitoring through behavioural changes such as improving inhaled-based medication adherence is of critical importance in maximising the efficiency of personalised medicine for asthma and COPD. Previous pilot trials have demonstrated the constructive impact of personalised asthma management plans for children [287] and adolescents [288]. The efficiency of such mhealth services for children can be further enhanced using interactive games such as the space-themed game, *Aspira* [289]. The benefits of mhealth for asthma management are not limited to inhaled medication adherence, and additional information, including lifestyle and environmental parameters, can be incorporated into the management plan. For example, GPS-based apps enable identifying triggers for an individual based on environmental measures including air temperature, humidity and potential allergens in the air; the latter can be extended to a link to an external weather server to notify the user of abrupt climate changes such as a sand storm [290]. Additionally, the app may incorporate the input from inertial sensors to track the exercise-based triggers. Besides accurate performance, the perceived user-friendliness of the asthma management app is of critical importance. To elevate the graphical design, Negar [291] investigated the features of the Graphical User Interface (GUI) and data presentation outlets by consulting professionals and end users. While the improved asthma outcome through personalised asthma self-monitoring plans reduces the number of in-person appointments, the e-visit feature of mhealth can be considered as a complementary cost containment strategy [46].

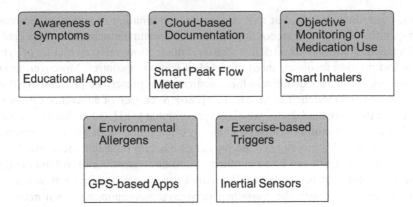

Fig. 3.8 The impact of mhealth solutions on asthma self-management

3.3.4 Objective Stress Monitoring

Mental health conditions, including stress-related disorders, are expected to be the second cause of disability by 2020 [292]. Anxiety and stress disorders are the most prevalent mental disorder and their prevalence is increasing over time [293]. According to Yerkes-Dodson Law, different levels of stress appear to have significant effects on behaviour [294]. While the low to moderate levels of stress have a constructive impact on the performance, the high stress level with devastating socioeconomic impact is considered a mental disorder [295, 296]. The stress disorder includes work-related stress, home stress and post-traumatic stress [297]. According to the WHO report in 2004, the post-traumatic stress disorder caused 3.5M DALYs lost globally; 0.5M and 3M in high-income countries and LMICs [298], respectively. Stress disorders also affect cognitive performance [299]. For instance, previous research has shown the correlation between driving with high levels of stress and crash involvement, because stress predisposes the driver to increased risk of road violation, cognitive lapses and errors [300–302]. Similarly, stress plays a considerable role in corporate health where its economic burden in the US is $300B per annum caused by a 46% increase in healthcare costs and reduced employee turnover, as well as legal costs and compensation [303]. mHealth offers a means to manage stress by monitoring its onset and delivering interventions. It has been confirmed that during mental stress, there is an increase in blood flow to several regions of the face, in particular the forehead region [304–306], while a meta-analysis of studies proved a correlation between stress and HRV [307]. Accordingly, either or both of HRV and the forehead thermal signal can be adopted as a biomarker for objective stress monitoring. A possible intervention to relieve stress is aromatherapy using the odorant lavender [308], which can be personalised through the application of novel detection and delivery mechanisms involving biosensors, fragrance technology and fashion. For example, eScent® [309] offers smart jewelleries that are linked wirelessly to sensors for monitoring the psychological status of the user and delivering the personalised wellbeing scents in response to a trigger by high levels of stress. An alternative intervention is through neurofeedback-based mobile meditation apps where a smart headset is used to measure the brain activity and offer immediate feedback to users for direct brain wave training which ultimately, leads to the management of stress [310, 311]. Also, the virtual reality option can be coupled with a smart headset to induce positive mood [312].

3.3.5 Drugs and Alcohol Consumption

Monitoring biothermal signals also enables extracting information about drug and alcohol consumption. The influence of the intake of medicaments such as paracetamol on the thermal-signals has been described in the literature [313–317]. However, there is no specific study on the effect of illicit drugs and therefore, a detailed investigation should be performed to define the effect of various drugs on facial thermal response. Moreover, intake of alcohol is associated with flushing due to skin vasodilation; for example, the temperature of the hand increased over the 9 min after consumption of 25 ml of 40% (alcohol by volume) whisky [318–321]. More research needs to be carried out to determine the effect of alcohol consumption on facial skin temperature and also evaluate the influence of factors such as the quantity of the alcohol, drinking habit and the duration of alcohol influence. This feature of alcohol intake empowers the police force to monitor the drivers of public transport and heavy vehicles, particularly those carrying explosive, flammable or toxic substances, and which eventually could enhance road safety, reduce the mortality rate and accidents involving heavy goods vehicles, buses and transportation of dangerous goods. The study on alcohol can be extended further to evaluate the influence of drinking water for the detection of dehydration [320]. This electrolyte disorder is more prevalent in elderly patients due to the deficiency of the thirst sensation [322]. The US National Health and Nutrition Examination Survey reported in 2005 that there was evidence of dehydration in 28% of the 70–90 year olds [323]. Dehydration is associated with an increase in the rate of readmission, hospital mortality, slow tissue recovery, pressure ulcers and developing chronic diseases, as well as significantly longer hospitalisation, particularly in intensive care units [324–326]. Thus, mhealth interventions to prevent dehydration could make a considerable contribution towards reducing healthcare costs (7–8.5% [327]) and improving health outcomes [324, 325].

3.3.6 Dermatology

Objective in vivo measurement of skin colour cues with high accuracy is needed in medical and cosmetic dermatology as it can be used an indicator of skin diseases and properties. There are several techniques for objective colour quantification: Full-range/narrow-band spectrophotometry, tristimulus colorimetery and digital photography. Hand-held reflectance spectroscopy-based instruments offer a highly accurate measurement [177, 328, 329]; however, they require significant financial investment [330], which could be prohibitive in many settings, and therefore digital photography, which is more readily accessible and less expensive to purchase and maintain, presents an attractive alternative. Digital photography is already used in dermatological practice to document cutaneous diseases and treatments [177]; however, it requires either a dedicated imaging laboratory or a reference colour plate to eliminate the effect of ambient lighting [328, 330]. A proposed smartphone-based imaging by the Lowe group allows a low-cost method that requires minimal training and is applicable in real-world settings with no need for accessories or a dedicated room to control ambient lighting [181]. This approach also promises clinicians value-added features and benefits for making decisions based on skin colour cues across the patient pathway from diagnosis to monitoring and treatment, such as: (1) Standardization of clinical diagnosis; (2) sensitive and reproducible assessment of disease severity and treatment efficacy; (3) precise grading and monitoring of colour changes; and, (4) optimisation of laser- and intense-pulsed-light-based treatment modalities to minimise risk of adverse effects and treatment discomfort. Moreover, the integration of this app and the healthcare provider's cloud enables: (1) implementation of a remote monitoring platform that allows individuals at risk to share their skin photographs taken at a third place in real world settings with clinicians for early, remote monitoring and detection; (2) development of a cloud-based photographic record of skin examination over time, which provides physicians the ability to follow and determine changes more efficiently; (3) a new way of networking and collaboration to share experiences of diagnosis and treatments with a peer group and also low-level clinicians can be authorised to perform at higher levels through real-time collaborations with experts and thereby deal with a shortage of physicians, particularly in underserved areas. Other specific benefits that can be driven from this approach are: (1) The Individual Typology Angle (°ITA) metric that provides an objective classification of skin colour types into 6 groups, ranging from very light that always burns and never tans to dark that is naturally pigmented black skin. This metric enables pre-evaluation of the Minimal Erythema Dose and also allows optimisation of treatment settings [331]; (2) Objective quantification of colour changes induced by erythema, tanning, topical corticosteroid preparation and long term haemodialysis, while also offering a metric to evaluate the efficacy of treatment. Moreover, skin colour change between summer and winter can be used to quantify changes in 25-hydroxyvitamin D [332]; (3) significant improvement in the performance of existing lesion segmentation algorithms in terms of accurately extracting skin lesion borders. Accordingly, it can help standardise melanoma studies by counting moles and tracking their size and density. This is of particular importance for variegated lesions such as acral lentiginous melanoma and lentigo maligna melanoma [179]; (4) conventional spectrophotometry-based colourimeters provide an estimate of average colour of the area surrounded by the aperture of the probe and thus lesions smaller than the aperture cannot be characterised separately, while this method enables image capture of a large tissue area and the colour measurements to be performed on any pixel of the digitally acquired and reproduced image. Thus, this mhealth instrument, free of calibration card and accessories, offers value-based services to dermatology. In terms of colour quantification, the accuracy of this approach is comparable to hand-held spectrophotometry-based techniques that cost between US$5000–15,000 per unit [177]. Moreover, the pre-processing steps can improve the performance of lesion segmentation especially in the case of complex mole patterns and hence reduces the need for biopsy [178] or expensive imaging technologies. Additionally, this approach promises clinicians value-added features and benefits for the treatment of acne, such as: (1) Standardisation of clinical diagnosis; (2) sensitive and reproducible assessment of disease severity and treatment efficacy; and (3) precise grading and monitoring of acne lesions.

3.3.7 Optometry and Ophthalmology

The application of mhealth in ophthalmology enables the assessment of visual acuity, colour vision, astigmatism, pupil size, Amsler grid test and fundus imaging (Fig. 3.9) [333, 334]. The inherent capabilities of mHealth has significant potential to tackle the socioeconomic burden of blindness due to uncorrected refractive errors which globally accounts for US$88.7–133B productivity loss. The prospect of smartphone-base eye care provides a cost-effective, ubiquitous platform to assess visual acuity, which is particularly valuable in developing countries where 87% of 2B people with uncorrected refractive errors live [335]. A review on mhealth apps in ophthalmology by Cheng et al. [336] showed a 12-fold increase in that the number of these apps in recent years. However, there are concerns regarding the clinical validation of these apps because only 68 out of 182 analysed apps had documented professional involvement. This demands a regulatory framework for dissemination of such apps while shortening the trial cycle for expedited delivery of these mhealth services to the primary stakeholders of healthcare [337]. Pathipati et al. [338] investigated the potential of automated smartphone-based optometry in emergency departments for staff members who are untrained in ophthalmology. Their study demonstrated that measuring the best-corrected visual acuity using the automated app offers a higher accuracy compared with the measurement obtained by non-ophthalmic staff of the emergency department using a standard Snellen chart. Accordingly, the average difference with the gold standard improved 0.147 logMAR (the logarithm of the Minimum Angle of Resolution; $p = 0.046$) which equals to more than a full line on a Snellen chart. Despite the potential of mhealth in testing visual acuity, the potential diversity in measurements across platforms, i.e. the near vision card and apps, due to the high contrast and brightness levels of smartphones should be considered [339].

The development of an inexpensive smartphone-based eye screening tool is also valuable for diagnosis of diabetic eye disease where a practical agreement with the clinical assessment is attainable. One of the common complications of diabetes is diabetic retinopathy (DR) with an estimated prevalence of 35% (~93M people globally in 2012) [340]. In 2003, DR globally accounted for ~2.5M of the estimated

Fig. 3.9 Examples of
the application of mhealth
solutions in optometry and
ophthalmology

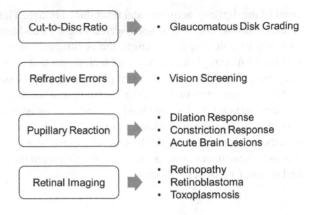

50M blindness cases in working age adults (20–60 years) [341] and the number is expected to triple by 2050 in countries such as the US [342]. The main contributor to the burden of DR is diagnosis at a stage that severe diabetic macular oedema and/or proliferative DR is developed [343, 344]. Hence, curbing the risk factor of DR demands addressing the lack of proper screening equipment mainly at primary care level, specifically in remote settings, for early diagnosis of DR during a long latent phase. Micheletti et al. [345] thoroughly reviewed the existing and under development portable technologies for DR screening that cost less than US$10K and weigh 5 lbs. Among these technologies, optical smartphone extension devices including SmartScope Pro [346] and iExaminer [347] have received FDA approval; however, their performance in terms of DR screening needs further improvement where the former offered a sensitivity and specificity of, respectively, 50–85% and 72–98% across different grading systems [345], and the latter has not been systematically evaluated [348]. There is a trend towards enhancing the performance characteristics of smartphone-based DR screening tools while optimising the engineering of accessories to minimise the related costs. Toy et al. [349] clinically assessed the performance of smartphone-based dilated fundus photography with that of standard comprehensive dilated eye examination and ultimately concluded that sensitivity and specificity of the smartphone-acquired fundus imaging for detecting moderate non-proliferative DR was 91% and 99%, respectively. In terms of cost, the fundus camera is about US$10K, whereas a smartphone and the 20 D lens is about US$500, implying that smartphone-based retinal imaging is more accessible for professionals in resource limited economies, e.g. Africa [196]. The total price of smartphone-based fundus examination can be further lowered by exploiting 3D printing for the development of extensions [350]. Adapting smartphone-based ocular diagnosis is equally advantageous in austere or warring environments, where there is a shortage or absence of ophthalmologists and optometrists where ocular injuries account for 13–22% of combat casualties and ≤32% in disaster scenarios [351, 352].

3.3.8 Cervical Cancer

According to the WHO, cervical cancer was the 4th most common cancer in women in 2012 with an estimated 528K incidences and accounting for 7.5% of all female cancer mortality [353]. The number of cervical cancer incidences over a four-decade time period in developed countries showed an 80% decrease [197]; a similar pattern was observed in lower middle income countries (LMICs) [354]. However, the prevalence in least developed nations soared [355]. On average, 9 out of 10 cases of cervical cancer death occur in less developed countries and result in ~85% of the relevant global burden [353]. The main contributor to this geographic variation in cervical cancer rates is access to screening, which can prevent the development of cancer through early detection and removal of premalignant lesions (cervical intraepithelial neoplasia; CIN). CIN is categorised based on the severity of dysplasia to CIN1 (low-grade), CIN2 and CIN3. CIN1 requires a repeat cervical screening test; however, treatment to remove abnormal cells (dyskaryosis) is recommended for types CIN2+. The strategies of the WHO to screen for cervical cancer include the Papanicolaou (Pap) test followed by a colposcopy in a positive Pap test, human papillomavirus (HPV) DNA test and visual inspection with 4% (v/v) acetic acid (VIA) or Lugol's iodine [356]. The Pap test and HPV DNA test demand access to robust healthcare infrastructures which are not available in countries with limited resources; for example, a conventional colposcope costs US$15K. There have been attempts to develop cost-effective colposcopy platforms: For example, a commercial product for cervical cancer screening has developed by MobileODT® [357] which offers a smartphone-based colposcopy for US$1800, which possesses a secure image transfer feature for a second opinion from a remote expert. However, this platform may not be affordable in the least developed nations. In this situation, the WHO recommends the VIA strategy [358], although the requirement for a trained mid-level healthcare professional might be a barrier. Moreover, the accuracy of VIA in randomised-controlled trials sounds less promising than cross-sectional studies [359]. Likewise, comparative studies demonstrated a considerable variability in CIN2+ detection rates [360, 361]. Improving quality assurance necessitates the development of an affordable imaging platform for low-resource settings. Stafl [362] proposed an alternative screening method for resource-limited nations, namely cervicography, which can be used by a non-physician health provider such as a midwife. Digital images of cervix before and after applying acetic acid or Lugol's iodine are obtained and sent to an expert for evaluation to improve the decision-making process. Clinical trials have demonstrated that the performance of cervicography in terms of sensitivity (for CIN2+) and specificity (to exclude CINs or cancer) is comparable with other methods [362–364]; however, there is a possibility of inflation of sensitivity of VIA [365]. The imaging technology in cervicography has progressed to enhance the quality digital images (cervigrams) [200]. In a clinical trial by Quinley et al. [198], a trained midwife used a mobile phone (Samsung SGH-U900; 5 MP) to capture and transmit cervigrams to a high-level physician, i.e. an expert gynaecologist, for remote diagnosis. Ricard-Gauthier et al. [199] evaluated the feasibility of capturing cervigrams using a high-quality smartphone (13 MP) for the detection of CIN2+ with an overall specificity of 79.2%. Urner et al. [366] studied the performance of smartphone-based cervicography with both acetic acid and Lugol's iodine for diagnosis of CIN2+ lesions which resulted in a higher sensitivity for acetic acid (94.1% vs. 78.8%) at the cost of a slightly lower specificity (56.4% vs. 50.4%).

3.3.9 Crohn's Disease

Crohn's disease is an inflammatory bowel disease which is a global challenge worldwide; however, the highest reported prevalence is reported in Europe and North America with 322 and 286 in 100,000, respectively [367]. However, this disease can go undetected due to limitations of existing technologies [368, 369]. An upper endoscopy stops around the duodenum [370] whereas 56% of Crohn's disease patients had lesions in their small bowel [371]. Examination of the small bowel is typically carried out using Computerised Tomography Enterography and Small Bowel Follow Through; however, these approaches causes exposure to X-ray and also have limitations in visualising the early stages of small bowel ulceration [372, 373]. PillCam™, as a smart medical device, address these drawbacks and enables non-invasive investigation of small bowel without exposing patients to radiation and through a patient-friendly approach [368, 374–377]. PillCam is also recommended for apparently healthy individuals because symptoms may not reflect the severity of diseases [378–380].

3.3.10 Pain Management

Pain represents substantial clinical and socioeconomic burden, with estimated prevalence of 8–60% [381]. For example, the indirect global cost of low back pain and osteoarthritis including lost income, reduced work productivity and the impact on GDP was 100M DALYS in 2010 [382]. In terms of the direct costs, namely "cost of care", an analysis from the Institute of Medicine in 2011 found that the average healthcare expenditure in the US on an individual suffering from pain is US$4516 higher than one without pain [383]. Still, there is not sufficient awareness regarding the magnitude of socioeconomic burden of pain, its impact on quality of life and the importance of its management. Hence, there is a need to implement well-validated, objective approaches for the assessment and management of pain [384]. Wearable neuro devices enable real-time monitoring of brain activity that can be analysed on a cloud-based platform to provide objective measurement of pain [385]. For instance, increased alpha and theta power at spontaneous EEG seems to be a clinical characteristic of individuals suffering from chronic pain [386]. Alternatively, PainQx [387] patented a quantitative electroencephalography (qEEG) approach to derive maps of brain functioning related to the sensation and perception of pain, namely "pain matrix", which offers a platform to quantify pain. This objective pain measurement is more reliable than subjective patient self-reports (i.e. Visual Analog Pain Scale, Numeric Rating Scale) that are highly prone to placebo responses [388]. Accordingly, smart headsets have the potential to allow accurate pain management which is critical to guide proper medical diagnosis, precise medicine selection, treatment, progress monitoring, real-time drug efficacy monitoring [16].

3.3.11 Rehabilitation

The global demographic change is expected to pose an increasing demand for functional rehabilitation in the future. The challenge is that rehabilitation therapies need to be carried out on a repetitive basis; for example, for muscle exercises it is typically 15–30 min, 2–5 times a week. This time consuming demand introduces a considerable pressure on healthcare systems economically and hence, healthcare providers are inclined to move rehabilitation outside hospital walls. A comprehensive review in Germany suggests innovative rehabilitation technologies have a considerable cost-saving potential by reducing 25–35% costs of rehabilitation with comparable effectiveness with inpatient care by introducing outpatient programmes at home [389]. Remote monitoring of sEMG (surface electromyography) as an mhealth solution empowers healthcare with therapeutic interventions to improve the rate of recovery and reduce the need for inpatient care. A matter of concern for remote rehabilitation considering its repetitive nature might be motivation problems with patients that can lead to low adherence to rehabilitation programmes and sub-optimal health outcomes. This challenge has been addressed by providing biofeedback through interactive games where the sEMG data provides required control commands for the game system. Previous studies have demonstrated coupling remote sEMG monitoring with interactive games in conjunction to regular physiotherapy sessions can enhance the involvement of patients in the treatment to improve their limitations [390–394]. Moreover, rehabilitation of individuals with sustain neurological impairments, such as acquired brain and spinal cord injuries, is achievable using sEMG-driven exoskeletons where the sEMG signals are monitored to trigger assistance to compensate lost functionality using, for example, neuro-fuzzy control systems and torque-estimation methods [395–400].

References

1. Kaniusas E (2012) Biomedical signals and sensors I: linking physiological phenomena and biosignals. Springer, Heidelberg
2. Huang M-C, Liu JJ, Xu W, Gu C, Li C, Sarrafzadeh M (2016) A self-calibrating radar sensor system for measuring vital signs. IEEE Trans Biomed Circuits Syst 10(2):352–363
3. Kranjec J, Beguš S, Geršak G, Drnovšek J (2014) Non-contact heart rate and heart rate variability measurements: a review. Biomed Signal Process Control 13:102–112

4. Dosinas A, Vaitkūnas M, Daunoras J (2006) Measurement of human physiological parameters in the systems of active clothing and wearable technologies. Elektron Elektrotech 71(7):77–82
5. Han T, Xiao X, Shi L, Canny J, Wang J (2015) Balancing accuracy and fun: designing camera based mobile games for implicit heart rate monitoring. In: 33rd Annual ACM Conference on Human Factors in Computing Systems, Seoul, South Korea, 18–23 April 2015
6. Abe E, Chigira H, Fujiwarai K, Yamakawa T, Kano M (2015) Heart rate monitoring by a pulse sensor embedded game controller. In: Asia-Pacific Signal and Information Processing Association Annual Summit and Conference, Hong Kong, China, 16–19 December 2015
7. Soares RT, Siqueira ES, Miura MA, e Silva TP, Castanho CD (2016) Biofeedback sensors in game telemetry research. http://www.sbgames.org/sbgames2016/downloads/anais/15748 2.pdf. Accessed Mar 2018
8. Sun Y, Thakor N (2016) Photoplethysmography revisited: from contact to noncontact, from point to imaging. IEEE Trans Biomed Eng 63(3):463–477
9. Katona J, Farkas I, Ujbanyi T, Dukan P, Kovari A (2014) Evaluation of the NeuroSky MindFlex EEG headset brain waves data. In: IEEE 12th International Symposium on Applied Machine Intelligence and Informatics, Herl'any, Slovakia, 23–25 January 2014
10. Siswoyo A, Arief Z, Sulistijono IA (2017) Application of artificial neural networks in modeling direction wheelchairs using neurosky mindset mobile (EEG) device. EMITTER 5(1):170–191
11. Tiwari K, Saini S (2015) Brain controlled robot using neurosky mindwave. JTASR 1(4):328–331
12. NeuroSky (2018) Brainwaves; not thoughts. http://neurosky.com/biosensors/eeg-sensor/. Accessed Mar 2018
13. Dave P (2015) Augmented reality start-up Daqri acquires smart headband maker Melon. Los Angeles Times. http://www.latimes.com/business/technology/la-fi-tn-daqri-melon-2015021 9-story.html. Accessed Mar 2018
14. MUSE (2018) Muse: the brain sensing headband. http://www.choosemuse.com/. Accessed Mar 2018
15. Emotive (2018) Emotive BrainWear. https://www.emotiv.com/. Accessed Mar 2018
16. Byrom B, Mc Carthy M, Schuleler P, Muehlhausen W (2018) Brain monitoring devices in neuroscience clinical research: the potential of remote monitoring using sensors, wearables and mobile devices. Clin Pharmacol Ther 104(1):59–71
17. Breuer T, Bruells CS, Rossaint R, Steffen H, Disselhorst-Klug C, Czaplik M, Zoremba N (2017) Acceleration sensors in abdominal wall position as a non-invasive approach to detect early breathing alterations induced by intolerance of increased airway resistance. J Cardiothorac Surg 12(1):96. https://doi.org/10.1186/s13019-017-0658-5
18. Aly H, Youssef M (2016) Zephyr: ubiquitous accurate multi-sensor fusion-based respiratory rate estimation using smartphones. In: The 35th Annual IEEE International Conference on Computer Communications, San Francisco, USA, 10–14 April 2016
19. Spiro (2018) Make your clothes smart. https://spire.io/. Accessed Mar 2018
20. ScienceDaily (2015) Wearable sensor clears path to long-term EKG, EMG monitoring. http://www.sciencedaily.com/releases/2015/01/150120102500.htm. Accessed Dec 2015
21. Gupta SKS, Mukherjee T, Venkatasubramanian KK (2013) Body area networks: safety, security, and sustainability. Cambridge University Press, UK
22. Vital Jacket (2015) Biodevices vital jacket—the future of heart monitoring. http://www.vital jacket.com/?page_id=156. Accessed Dec 2015
23. Hornyak T (2013) Undershirt monitors heart rate with wearable electrodes. http://www.cnet. com/news/undershirt-monitors-heart-rate-with-wearable-electrodes/. Accessed Dec 2015
24. Paradiso R, Loriga G, Taccini N, Pacelli M, Orselli R (2004) Wearable system for vital signs monitoring. Stud Health Technol Inform 108:253–259
25. Pandian P, Mohanavelu K, Safeer K, Kotresh T, Shakunthala D, Gopal P, Padaki V (2008) Smart Vest: wearable multi-parameter remote physiological monitoring system. Med Eng Phys 30(4):466–477

26. Di Rienzo M, Racca V, Rizzo F, Bordoni B, Parati G, Castiglioni P, Meriggi P, Ferratini M (2013) Evaluation of a textile-based wearable system for the electrocardiogram monitoring in cardiac patients. Europace 15(4):607–612

27. Morrison T, Silver J, Otis B (2014) A single-chip encrypted wireless 12-lead ECG smart shirt for continuous health monitoring. In: Symposium on VLSI Circuits Digest of Technical Papers, Honolulu, USA, 10–13 June 2014

28. HealthWatch (2014) hWear Digital Garments. http://www.personal-healthwatch.com/hwear-health-sensing-garments.aspx. Accessed Dec 2015

29. Jones, MT, Martin, TL (2009) Hardware and Software Architectures for Electronic Textiles. In: Cho G (ed) Smart clothing: technology and applications. CRC Press, USA

30. Redmond S, Ee Y, Basilakis J, Celler B, Lovell N (2009) ECG recording and rhythm analysis for distributed health care environments. In: Acharya UR, Tamura T, Ng EYK, Min LC, Sure JS (eds) Distributed diagnosis and home healthcare. American Scientific, USA

31. Srikureja W, Darbar D, Reeder GS (2000) Tremor-induced ECG artifact mimicking ventricular tachycardia. Circulation 102(11):1337–1338

32. Edelberg R (1973) Local electrical response of the skin to deformation. J Appl Physiol 34(3):334–340

33. Finni T, Hu M, Kettunen P, Vilavuo T, Cheng S (2007) Measurement of EMG activity with textile electrodes embedded into clothing. Physiol Meas 28(11):1405

34. Myontec (2018) MBODY AllSport 6 Channel. https://www.myontec.com/products/mbody/. Accessed Mar 2018

35. Düking P, Hotho A, Holmberg H-C, Fuss FK, Sperlich B (2016) Comparison of non-invasive individual monitoring of the training and health of athletes with commercially available wearable technologies. Front Physiol 7:71. https://doi.org/10.3389/fphys.2016.00071

36. De Luca CJ (1997) The use of surface electromyography in biomechanics. J Appl Biomech 13(2):135–163

37. Belbasis A, Fuss FK (2015) Development of next-generation compression apparel. Proc Tech 20:85–90

38. Colyer SL, McGuigan PM (2018) Textile electrodes embedded in clothing: a practical alternative to traditional surface electromyography when assessing muscle excitation during functional movements. J Sports Sci Med 17(1):101–109

39. Hakonen M, Piitulainen H, Visala A (2015) Current state of digital signal processing in myoelectric interfaces and related applications. Biomed Signal Process Control 18:334–359

40. Burgess SW, Wilson SS, Cooper DM, Sly PD, Devadason SG (2006) In vitro evaluation of an asthma dosing device: the smart-inhaler. Resp Med 100(5):841–845

41. Perez C (2015) Smart inhalers and the future of respiratory health management: smart inhalers are part of a new wave of digital technology designed to improve the management of lung diseases. In: RT for Decision Makers in Respiratory Care 28(10):10–14. http://www.rtmagazine.com/2015/10/smart-inhalers-future-respiratory-health-management/. Accessed Mar 2018

42. Chen C-C, Liu Y-J, Sung G-N, Yang C-C, Wu C-M, Huang C-M (2015) Smart electronic dose counter for pressurized metered dose inhaler. In: IEEE Biomedical Circuits and Systems Conference, Atlanta, USA, 22–24 October 2015

43. Furst SJ, Seelecke S (2014) Fabrication and characterization of a dual-joint smart inhaler nozzle actuated by embedded SMA wires. Smart Mater Struct 23(3):035008

44. Howard S, Lang A, Sharples S, Shaw D (2017) See I told you I was taking it!—attitudes of adolescents with asthma towards a device monitoring their inhaler use: implications for future design. Appl Ergon 58:224–237

45. Kikidis D, Konstantinos V, Tzovaras D, Usmani OS (2016) The digital asthma patient: the history and future of inhaler based health monitoring devices. J Aerosol Med Pulm Drug Deliv 29(3):219–232

46. Asthma UK (2017) Smart asthma: real-world implementation of connected devices in the UK to reduce asthma attacks. https://www.asthma.org.uk/globalassets/get-involved/external-affairs-campaigns/publications/smart-asthma/auk_smartasthma_feb2017.pdf. Accessed Mar 2018

47. Chamberlain D, Jimenez-Galindo A, Fletcher RR, Kodgule R (2016) Applying augmented reality to enable automated and low-cost data capture from medical devices. In: Proceedings of the 8th International Conference on Information and Communication Technologies and Development, Ann Arbor, USA, 3–6 June 2016

48. Kassem A, Hamad M, El-Moucary C, Neghawi E, Jaoude GB, Merhej C (2013) Asthma care apps. In: 2nd International Conference on Advances in Biomedical Engineering, Tripoli, Lebanon, 11–13 September 2013

49. Kassem A, Hamad M, El Moucary C (2015) A smart spirometry device for asthma diagnosis. In: 37th Annual International Conference of the IEEE Engineering in Medicine and Biology Society, Milan, Italy, 25–29 August 2015

50. Carspecken CW, Arteta C, Clifford GD (2013) TeleSpiro: a low-cost mobile spirometer for resource-limited settings. In: IEEE Point-of-Care Healthcare Technologies, Bangalore, India, 16–18 January 2013

51. Gupta S, Chang P, Anyigbo N, Sabharwal A (2011) mobileSpiro: accurate mobile spirometry for self-management of asthma. In: Proceedings of the First ACM Workshop on Mobile Systems, Applications, and Services for Healthcare, Seattle, USA, 1 November 2011

52. Bumatay A, Chan R, Lauher K, Kwan AM, Stoltz T, Delplanque J-P, Kenyon NJ, Davis CE (2012) Coupled mobile phone platform with peak flow meter enables real-time lung function assessment. IEEE Sens J 12(3):685–691

53. Natarajan S, Castner J, Titus A (2016) Smart phone-based peak expiratory flow meter. Electron Lett 52(11):904–905

54. HealthUp (2017) MySpiroo. http://www.myspiroo.com/#About. Accessed Mar 2018

55. Smart Peak Flow™ (2017) Asthma control in your pocket. http://www.smartpeakflow.com/. Accessed Mar 2018

56. MIR Medical International Research (2017) SMARTONE®. https://www.spirometry.com/en g/products/smartone.asp. Accessed Mar 2018

57. Wing (2017) Don't let COPD land you in the hospital. https://mywing.io/. Accessed Mar 2018

58. Schneider AM (2015) Personalized asthma medication. Dissertation, Umeå University

59. Blake WK (1986) Mechanics of flow-induced sound and vibration: complex flow-structure interactions. Academic Press, USA

60. Hardin J, Patterson J (1979) Monitoring the state of the human airways by analysis of respiratory sound. Acta Astronaut 6(9):1137–1151

61. Luisada A (1964) The areas of auscultation and the two main heart sounds. Med Times 92:8–11

62. Sprague HB, Ongley PA (1954) The clinical value of phonocardiography. Circulation 9(1):127–134

63. Littmann® M Electronic Stethoscopes (2015) 3M™ Littmann®. https://www.littmann.com/3 M/en_US/littmann-stethoscopes/products/~/3M-Littmann-Stethoscopes/Electronic-Stethosc opes/?N=5142935+8711017+8727094+3294857497&rt=r3. Accessed Dec 2016

64. Jatupaiboon N, Pan-Ngum S, Israsena P (2010) Electronic stethoscope prototype with adaptive noise cancellation. In: 8th International Conference on ICT and Knowledge Engineering, Bangkok, Thailand, 24–25 November 2010

65. Ghavami M (1998) Adaptive line enhancement using a parallel iir filter with a step-by-step algorithm. Int J Eng 11(2):73

66. Lakhe A, Sodhi I, Warrier J, Sinha V (2016) Development of digital stethoscope for telemedicine. J Med Eng Technol 40(1):20–24

67. Gnitecki J, Moussavi ZM (2007) Separating heart sounds from lung sounds. IEEE Eng Med Biol Mag 26(1):20–29

68. Gupta S, Pandey S, Jiavana FK (2016) Low noise electronic stethoscope. Adv Nat Appl Sci 10(14):52–58

69. Das D, Banerjee R, Choudhury AD, Deshpande P, Shah N, Date V, Pal A, Mandana KM (2017) Noise detection in smartphone phonocardiogram. In: 2017 IEEE International Conference on Acoustics, Speech and Signal Processing, New Orleans, USA, 5–9 March 2017

70. Das D, Banerjee R, Choudhury AD, Bhattacharya S, Deshpande P, Pal A, Mandana KM (2017) Novel features from autocorrelation and spectrum to classify Phonocardiogram quality. In: 39th Annual International Conference of the IEEE Engineering in Medicine and Biology Society, Seogwipo, South Korea, 11–15 July 2017

71. Springer DB, Brennan T, Zuhlke LJ, Abdelrahman HY, Ntusi N, Clifford GD, Mayosi BM, Tarassenko L (2014) Signal quality classification of mobile phone-recorded phonocardiogram signals. In: IEEE International Conference on Acoustics, Speech and Signal Processing, Florence, Italy, 4–9 May 2014

72. Springer DB, Brennan T, Ntusi N, Abdelrahman HY, Zühlke LJ, Mayosi BM, Tarassenko L, Clifford GD (2016) Automated signal quality assessment of mobile phone-recorded heart sound signals. J Med Eng Technol 40(7–8):342–355

73. Kumar D, Carvalho P, Antunes M, Paiva R, Henriques J (2011) Noise detection during heart sound recording using periodicity signatures. Physiol Meas 32(5):599–618

74. Thinklabs (2017) Thinklabs One Digital Stethoscope. http://www.thinklabs.com/one-digital-stethoscope. Accessed Aug 2017

75. HD Medical (2017) ViScope MD. http://hdmedicalgroup.com/our-products/viscope-md/. Accessed Aug 2017

76. Sinharay A, Ghosh D, Deshpande P, Alam S, Banerjee R, Pal A (2016) Smartphone based digital stethoscope for connected health—a direct acoustic coupling technique. In: IEEE 1st International Conference on Connected Health: Applications, Systems and Engineering Technologies, Washington, USA, 27–29 June 2016

77. Aguilera-Astudillo C, Chavez-Campos M, Gonzalez-Suarez A, Garcia-Cordero JL (2016) A low-cost 3-D printed stethoscope connected to a smartphone. In: 38th Annual International Conference of Engineering in Medicine and Biology Society, Orlando, USA, 16–20 August 2016

78. Gauthier D, Akay YM, Paden RG, Pavlicek W, Fortuin FD, Sweeney JK, Lee RW, Akay M (2007) Spectral analysis of heart sounds associated with coronary occlusions. In: 6th International Special Topic Conference on Information Technology Applications in Biomedicine, Tokyo, Japan, 8–11 November 2007

79. Schmidt SE, Hansen J, Zimmermann H, Hammersh D, Toft E, Struijk JJ (2011) Coronary artery disease and low frequency heart sound signatures. In: Computing in Cardiology, Hangzhou, China, 18–21 September 2011

80. Huiying L, Sakari L, Iiro H (1997) A heart sound segmentation algorithm using wavelet decomposition and reconstruction. In: 19th Annual International Conference of the IEEE Engineering in Medicine and Biology Society, Chicago, USA, 30 October–2 November 1997

81. Harsola A, Thale S, Panse M (2011) Low cost digital stethoscope for heart sounds. In: Proceedings of the International Conference & Workshop on Emerging Trends in Technology, Mumbai, India, 25–26 February 2011

82. Herzig J, Bickel A, Eitan A, Intrator N (2015) Monitoring cardiac stress using features extracted from S1 heart sounds. IEEE Trans Biomed Eng 62(4):1169–1178

83. Ahlstrom C, Hult P, Rask P, Karlsson J-E, Nylander E, Dahlström U, Ask P (2006) Feature extraction for systolic heart murmur classification. Ann Biomed Eng 34(11):1666–1677

84. Jabbari S, Ghassemian H (2011) Modeling of heart systolic murmurs based on multivariate matching pursuit for diagnosis of valvular disorders. Comput Biol Med 41(9):802–811

85. Maglogiannis I, Loukis E, Zafiropoulos E, Stasis A (2009) Support vectors machine-based identification of heart valve diseases using heart sounds. Comput Methods Programs Biomed 95(1):47–61

86. Huang NE, Shen Z, Long SR, Wu MC, Shih HH, Zheng Q, Yen N-C, Tung CC, Liu HH (1998) The empirical mode decomposition and the Hilbert spectrum for nonlinear and non-stationary time series analysis. In: Proceedings of the Royal Society of London A: Mathematical, Physical and Engineering Sciences. The Royal Society Publishing, UK

87. Sun S (2015) An innovative intelligent system based on automatic diagnostic feature extraction for diagnosing heart diseases. Knowl-Based Syst 75:224–238

88. Tseng Y-L, Ko P-Y, Jaw F-S (2012) Detection of the third and fourth heart sounds using Hilbert-Huang transform. Biomed Eng Online 11:8. https://doi.org/10.1186/1475-925X-11-8

89. Kumar D, Carvalho P, Antunes M, Henriques J, e Melo AS, Habetha J (2008) Heart murmur recognition and segmentation by complexity signatures. In: 30th Annual International Conference of the IEEE Engineering in Medicine and Biology Society, Vancouver, Canada, 20–25 August 2008

90. Yuenyong S, Nishihara A, Kongprawechnon W, Tungpimolrut K (2011) A framework for automatic heart sound analysis without segmentation. Biomed Eng Online 10:13. https://doi.org/10.1186/1475-925X-10-13

91. Deng S-W, Han J-Q (2016) Towards heart sound classification without segmentation via autocorrelation feature and diffusion maps. Future Gener Comput Syst 60:13–21

92. Banerjee R, Choudhury AD, Deshpande P, Bhattacharya S, Pal A, Mandana K (2017) A robust dataset-agnostic heart disease classifier from Phonocardiogram. In: 39th Annual International Conference of the IEEE Engineering in Medicine and Biology Society, Seogwipo, South Korea, 11–15 July 2017

93. iHealth Labs (2018) iHealth Sense. https://ihealthlabs.com/blood-pressure-monitors/wireless-blood-pressure-wrist-monitor/. Accessed Mar 2018

94. McElhearn K (2014) Withings wireless blood pressure monitor review: HealthKit compatibility doesn't add much. https://www.macworld.com/article/2851095/withings-wireless-blood-pressure-monitor-review-healthkit-compatibility-doesnt-add-much.html. Accessed Mar 2018

95. Balestrieri E, Rapuano S (2009) Advances in biomedical sensing, measurements, instrumentation and systems. In: Lay-Ekuakille A, Mukhopadhyay SC (eds) Lecture notes in electrical engineering, vol 55. Springer, Heidelberg

96. Haridy R (2017) Pocket-sized, affordably-priced ultrasound connects to an iPhone. https://newatlas.com/butterfly-iq-smartphone-ultrasound/51962/. Accessed Dec 2017

97. MobiSante (2018) MobiSante smartphone ultrasound: the MobiUS SP1 system. http://www.mobisante.com/products/product-overview/. Accessed Mar 2018

98. Philips (2018) Lumify exceptional portable ultrasound from your smart device. https://www.lumify.philips.com/web/. Accessed Mar 2018

99. Butterfly Network (2018) Butterfly meet iQ. https://www.butterflynetwork.com/. Accessed Mar 2018

100. Clarius (2018) Wireless portable ultrasound. https://www.clarius.com/. Accessed Mar 2018

101. PillCam (2018) PillCam SB capsule. https://www.pillcamcrohns.com/. Accessed Mar 2018

102. Medtronic (2018) SmartPill motility testing system. http://www.medtronic.com/covidien/en-us/products/motility-testing/smartpill-motility-testing-system.html. Accessed Mar 2018

103. Nakashima H, Aghajan H, Augusto JC (eds) (2009) Handbook of ambient intelligence and smart environments. Springer, US

104. Kim K-S, Yoon T-H, Lee J-W, Kim D-J (2009) Interactive toothbrushing education by a smart toothbrush system via 3D visualization. Comput Methods Programs Biomed 96(2):125–132

105. Marcon M, Sarti A, Tubaro S (2016) Toothbrush motion analysis to help children learn proper tooth brushing. Comput Vis Image Underst 148:34–45

106. Marcon M, Sarti A, Tubaro S (2016) Smart toothbrushes: inertial measurement sensors fusion with visual tracking. In: European Conference on Computer Vision, Amsterdam, Netherlands, 8–16 October 2016

107. Kolibree (2014) Kolibree toothbrush. https://www.kolibree.com/en/. Accessed Dec 2017

108. Oral-B (2017) Pro 5000 with bluetooth connectivity electric rechargeable toothbrush. https://oralb.com/en-us/products/pro-5000-electric-toothbrush-with-smartguide-bluetooth. Accessed Dec 2017

109. Prophix (2017) Prophix smart toothbrush by onvi. https://www.getprophix.com/. Accessed Dec 2017

110. PlayBrush (2017) PlayBrush—your smart toothbrush. https://www.playbrush.com/en/. Accessed Dec 2017

111. Philips Sonicare (2017) FlexCare platinum connected. https://www.usa.philips.com/c-m-pe/electric-toothbrushes/flexcare-platinum/connected. Accessed Dec 2017
112. BleepBleeps (2017) Benjamin brush smart music toothbrush. https://bleepbleeps.com/pages/benjamin-brush-smart-music-toothbrush. Accessed Dec 2017
113. Bacquet and Riemenschneider (2017) Next Generation IoT Platforms. In: Vermesan O, Bacquet J (eds) Cognitive hyperconnected digital transformation: internet of things intelligence evolution. River Publishers, Denmark
114. Balakrishnan G, Durand F, Guttag J (2013) Detecting pulse from head motions in video. In: IEEE Conference on Computer Vision and Pattern Recognition, Portland, USA, 23–28 June 2013
115. Shan L, Yu M (2013) Video-based heart rate measurement using head motion tracking and ICA. In: 6th International Congress on Image and Signal Processing, Hangzhou, China, 16–18 December 2013
116. Irani R, Nasrollahi K, Moeslund TB (2014) Improved pulse detection from head motions using DCT. In: International Conference on Computer Vision Theory and Applications, Lisbon, Portugal, 5–8 January 2014
117. Sikdar A, Behera SK, Dogra DP (2016) Computer-vision-guided human pulse rate estimation: a review. IEEE Rev Biomed Eng 9:91–105
118. Hassan M, Malik A, Fofi D, Saad N, Karasfi B, Ali Y, Meriaudeau F (2017) Heart rate estimation using facial video: a review. Biomed Signal Process Control 38:346–360
119. Wieringa FP, Mastik F, van der Steen AF (2005) Contactless multiple wavelength photoplethysmographic imaging: a first step toward "SpO2 camera" technology. Ann Biomed Eng 33(8):1034–1041
120. Stankevich E, Paramonov I, Timofeev I (2012) Mobile phone sensors in health applications. In: 12th Conference of Open Innovations Association, Oulu, Finland, 5–9 November 2012
121. Pawankiattikun V, Kondo T (2014) A method for contact-free heart rate measurement on a video sequence using simulink. In: 7th Biomedical Engineering International Conference, Fukuoka, Japan, 26–28 November 2014
122. Pursche T, Krajewski J, Moeller R (2012) Video-based heart rate measurement from human faces. In: IEEE International Conference on Consumer Electronics, Las Vegas, USA, 13–16 January 2012
123. Lee K-Z, Hung P-C, Tsai L-W (2012) Contact-free heart rate measurement using a camera. In: 9th Conference on Computer and Robot Vision, Toronto, Canada, 28–30 November 2012
124. Verkruysse W, Svaasand LO, Nelson JS (2008) Remote plethysmographic imaging using ambient light. Opt Express 16(26):21434–21445
125. Jonathan E, Leahy M (2010) Investigating a smartphone imaging unit for photoplethysmography. Physiol Meas 31(11):N79–N83
126. Jonathan E, Leahy MJ (2011) Cellular phone-based photoplethysmographic imaging. J Biophotonics 4(5):293–296
127. Kwon S, Kim H, Park KS (2012) Validation of heart rate extraction using video imaging on a built-in camera system of a smartphone. In: Annual International Conference of the IEEE Engineering in Medicine and Biology Society, San Diego, USA, 28 August–1 September 2012
128. Al-Naji A, Perera AG, Chahl J (2017) Remote monitoring of cardiorespiratory signals from a hovering unmanned aerial vehicle. Biomed Eng Online 16(1):101. https://doi.org/10.1186/s12938-017-0395-y
129. Li X, Chen J, Zhao G, Pietikainen M (2014) Remote heart rate measurement from face videos under realistic situations. In: IEEE Conference on Computer Vision and Pattern Recognition, Columbus, USA, 23–28 June 2014
130. Kumar M, Veeraraghavan A, Sabharwal A (2015) DistancePPG: robust non-contact vital signs monitoring using a camera. Biomed Opt Express 6(5):1565–1588
131. Huelsbusch M (2008) An image-based functional method for opto-electronic detection of skin-perfusion. Dissertation, RWTH Aachen University

132. Lewandowska M, Rumiński J, Kocejko T, Nowak J (2011) Measuring pulse rate with a webcam—a non-contact method for evaluating cardiac activity. In: Federated Conference on Computer Science and Information Systems, Szczecin, Poland, 18–21 September 2011

133. Poh M-Z, McDuff DJ, Picard RW (2011) Advancements in noncontact, multiparameter physiological measurements using a webcam. IEEE Trans Biomed Eng 58(1):7–11

134. Poh M-Z, McDuff DJ, Picard RW (2010) Non-contact, automated cardiac pulse measurements using video imaging and blind source separation. Opt Express 18(10):10762–10774

135. Rouast PV, Adam MT, Chiong R, Cornforth D, Lux E (2017) Remote heart rate measurement using low-cost RGB face video: a technical literature review. Front Comput Sci. https://doi.org/10.1007/s11704-016-6243-6

136. Yu Y-P, Kwan B-H, Lim C-L, Wong S-L, Raveendran P (2013) Video-based heart rate measurement using short-time Fourier transform. In: International Symposium on Intelligent Signal Processing and Communications Systems, Naha, Japan, 12–15 November 2013

137. Wei L, Tian Y, Wang Y, Ebrahimi T, Huang T (2012) Automatic webcam-based human heart rate measurements using laplacian eigenmap. In: Lee KM, Matsushita Y, Rehg JM, Hu Z (eds) Computer Vision—ACCV 2012. ACCV 2012. Lecture notes in computer science, vol 7725. Springer, Heidelberg

138. Li M-C, Lin Y-H (2015) A real-time non-contact pulse rate detector based on smartphone. In: International Symposium on Next-Generation Electronics, Taipei, Taiwan, 4–6 May 2015

139. McDuff D, Gontarek S, Picard RW (2014) Improvements in remote cardiopulmonary measurement using a five band digital camera. IEEE Trans Biomed Eng 61(10):2593–2601

140. Lam A, Kuno Y (2015) Robust heart rate measurement from video using select random patches. In: IEEE International Conference on Computer Vision, Santiago, Chile, 7–13 December 2015

141. Wu H-Y (2012) Eulerian video processing and medical applications. Dissertation, Massachusetts Institute of Technology

142. Datcu D, Cidota M, Lukosch S, Rothkrantz L (2013) Noncontact automatic heart rate analysis in visible spectrum by specific face regions. In: Proceedings of the 14th International Conference on Computer Systems and Technologies, Ruse, Bulgaria, 28–29 June 2013

143. Fallet S, Moser V, Braun F, Vesin J-M (2016) Imaging photoplethysmography: what are the best locations on the face to estimate heart rate? In: Computing in Cardiology Conference, Vancouver, Canada, 11–14 September 2016

144. Blackford EB, Estepp JR, Piasecki AM, Bowers MA, Klosterman SL (2016) Long-range non-contact imaging photoplethysmography: cardiac pulse wave sensing at a distance. In: Optical Diagnostics and Sensing XVI: Toward Point-of-Care Diagnostics, San Francisco, USA, 13–18 February 2016

145. Sun Y, Papin C, Azorin-Peris V, Kalawsky R, Greenwald S, Hu S (2012) Use of ambient light in remote photoplethysmographic systems: comparison between a high-performance camera and a low-cost webcam. J Biomed Opt 17(3):0370051–03700510

146. Kong L, Zhao Y, Dong L, Jian Y, Jin X, Li B, Feng Y, Liu M, Liu X, Wu H (2013) Non-contact detection of oxygen saturation based on visible light imaging device using ambient light. Opt Express 21(15):17464–17471

147. Feng L, Po L-M, Xu X, Li Y, Ma R (2015) Motion-resistant remote imaging photoplethysmography based on the optical properties of skin. IEEE Trans Circuits Syst Video Technol 25(5):879–891

148. Henriques JF, Caseiro R, Martins P, Batista J (2012) Exploiting the circulant structure of tracking-by-detection with kernels. In: 12th European Conference on Computer Vision, Florence, Italy, 7–13 October 2012

149. Haan Gd, Jeanne V (2013) Robust pulse rate from chrominance-based rPPG. IEEE Trans Biomed Eng 60(10):2878–2886

150. Wang W, Stuijk S, De Haan G (2015) Exploiting spatial redundancy of image sensor for motion robust rPPG. IEEE Trans Biomed Eng 62(2):415–425

151. Haan Gd, Van Leest A (2014) Improved motion robustness of remote-PPG by using the blood volume pulse signature. Physiol Meas 35(9):1913

152. Wang W, Stuijk S, De Haan G (2016) A novel algorithm for remote photoplethysmography: spatial subspace rotation. IEEE Trans Biomed Eng 63(9):1974–1984
153. Fan X (2017) Scalable teaching and learning via intelligent user interfaces. Dissertation, University of Pittsburgh
154. Arandjelovic O (2012) Gradient edge map features for frontal face recognition under extreme illumination changes. In: 23rd British Machine Vision Conference, Surrey, UK, 3–7 September 2012
155. Bal U (2015) Non-contact estimation of heart rate and oxygen saturation using ambient light. Biomed Opt Express 6(1):86–97
156. McDuff D, Gontarek S, Picard RW (2014) Remote detection of photoplethysmographic systolic and diastolic peaks using a digital camera. IEEE Trans Biomed Eng 61(12):2948–2954
157. Xu S, Sun L, Rohde GK (2014) Robust efficient estimation of heart rate pulse from video. Biomed Opt Express 5(4):1124–1135
158. Scully CG, Lee J, Meyer J, Gorbach AM, Granquist-Fraser D, Mendelson Y, Chon KH (2012) Physiological parameter monitoring from optical recordings with a mobile phone. IEEE Trans Biomed Eng 59(2):303–306
159. Chong JW, Esa N, McManus DD, Chon KH (2015) Arrhythmia discrimination using a smart phone. IEEE J Biomed Health Inform 19(3):815–824
160. McManus DD, Lee J, Maitas O, Esa N, Pidikiti R, Carlucci A, Harrington J, Mick E, Chon KH (2013) A novel application for the detection of an irregular pulse using an iPhone 4S in patients with atrial fibrillation. Heart Rhythm 10(3):315–319
161. Lee J, Reyes BA, McManus DD, Maitas O, Chon KH (2013) Atrial fibrillation detection using an iPhone 4S. IEEE Trans Biomed Eng 60(1):203–206
162. Huang S-C, Hung P-H, Hong C-H, Wang H-M (2014) A new image blood pressure sensor based on PPG, RRT, BPTT, and harmonic balancing. IEEE Sens J 14(10):3685–3692
163. Rea MS (ed) (2000) The IESNA lighting handbook: reference and application. Illuminating Engineering Society of North America, USA
164. Tarassenko L, Villarroel M, Guazzi A, Jorge J, Clifton D, Pugh C (2014) Non-contact video-based vital sign monitoring using ambient light and auto-regressive models. Physiol Meas 35(5):807–813
165. Belhumeur PN, Kriegman DJ (1998) What is the set of images of an object under all possible illumination conditions? Int J Comput Vision 28(3):245–260
166. Georghiades AS, Belhumeur PN, Kriegman DJ (2000) From few to many: generative models for recognition under variable pose and illumination. In: 4th IEEE International Conference on Automatic Face and Gesture Recognition, Grenoble, France, 28–30 March 2000
167. Riklin-Raviv T, Shashua A (1999) The quotient image: class based re-rendering and recognition with varying illuminations. IEEE Trans Pattern Anal Mach Intell 23(2):129–139
168. Blanz V, Romdhani S, Vetter T (2002) Face identification across different poses and illuminations with a 3d morphable model. In: 5th IEEE International Conference on Automatic Face and Gesture Recognition, Washington, USA, 21 May 2002
169. Chen D-Y, Wang J-J, Lin K-Y, Chang H-H, Wu H-K, Chen Y-S, Lee S-Y (2015) Image sensor-based heart rate evaluation from face reflectance using Hilbert-Huang transform. IEEE Sens J 15(1):618–627
170. Lee D, Kim J, Kwon S, Park K (2015) Heart rate estimation from facial photoplethysmography during dynamic illuminance changes. In: 37th Annual International Conference of the IEEE Engineering in Medicine and Biology Society, Milan, Italy, 25–29 August 2015
171. Cheng J, Chen X, Xu L, Wang ZJ (2016) Illumination variation-resistant video-based heart rate measurement using joint blind source separation and ensemble empirical mode decomposition. IEEE J Biomed Health Inform 21(5):1422–1433
172. Blackford EB, Estepp JR (2015) Effects of frame rate and image resolution on pulse rate measured using multiple camera imaging photoplethysmography. In: Medical Imaging 2015: Biomedical Applications in Molecular, Structural, and Functional Imaging, Orlando, USA, 21–26 February 2015

173. McDuff DJ, Blackford EB, Estepp JR (2017) The impact of video compression on remote cardiac pulse measurement using imaging photoplethysmography. In: 12th IEEE International Conference on Automatic Face & Gesture Recognition, Washington, USA, 30 May–3 June 2017

174. Wang W, den Brinker AC, Stuijk S, de Haan G (2017) Algorithmic principles of remote PPG. IEEE Trans Biomed Eng 64(7):1479–1491

175. McDuff DJ, Estepp JR, Piasecki AM, Blackford EB (2015) A survey of remote optical photoplethysmographic imaging methods. In: 37th Annual International Conference of the IEEE Engineering in Medicine and Biology Society, Milan, Italy, 25–29 August 2015

176. Daw W, Kingshott R, Saatchi R, Burke D, Holloway A, Travis J, Evans R, Jones A, Hughes B, Elphick H (2016) Medical devices for measuring respiratory rate in children. J Adv Biomed Eng Technol 3:21–27

177. Everett JS, Budescu M, Sommers MS (2012) Making sense of skin color in clinical care. Clin Nurs Res 21(4):495–516

178. O'Donnell AT, Kim CC (2012) Update and clinical use of imaging technologies for pigmented lesions of the skin. Semin Cutan Med Surg 31(1):38–44

179. Rathore S, Kower M, Kumar TS (2013) Colour and contrast enhancement for improved skin lesion segmentation using retinex theory. IJERT 2(7):2450–2456

180. Witmer WK, Lebovitz PJ (2012) Clinical photography in the dermatology practice. Semin Cutan Med Surg 31(3):191–199

181. Khalili Moghaddam G (2016) Quantitative measurements on holographic grating sensors for point-of-care diagnostics. Dissertation, University of Cambridge

182. Garg SJ (2016) Applicability of smartphone-based screening programs. JAMA ophthalmol 134(2):158–159

183. Giardini ME, Livingstone IA, Jordan S, Bolster NM, Peto T, Burton M, Bastawrous A (2014) A smartphone based ophthalmoscope. In: 36th Annual International Conference of the IEEE Engineering in Medicine and Biology Society, Chicago, USA, 26–30 August 2014

184. Bastawrous A, Leak C, Howard F, Kumar V (2012) Validation of near eye tool for refractive assessment (NETRA)—Pilot study. J Mob Technol Med 1(3):6–16

185. Gaiser H, Moore B, Pamplona V, Solaka N, Schafran D, Merrill D, Sharpe N, Geringer J, Raskar R (2013) Comparison of a novel cell phone-based refraction technique (Netra-G) with subjective refraction. Invest Ophth Vis Sci 54(15):2340

186. Ciuffreda KJ, Rosenfield M (2015) Evaluation of the SVOne: a handheld, smartphone-based autorefractor. Optom Vision Sci 92(12):1133–1139

187. Fink W, Garcia K, Tarbell M (2016) Smartphone-based head-mounted binocular high-speed pupillometer. In: Annual Meeting of the Association for Research in Vision and Ophthalmology, Seattle, USA, 1–5 May

188. Fink W, Tarbell M (2015) Smart ophthalmics: a smart service platform for tele-ophthalmology. Invest Ophth Vis Sci 56(7):4110

189. Park JG, Moon CT, Park DS, Song SW (2015) Clinical utility of an automated pupillometer in patients with acute brain lesion. J Korean Neurosurg Soc 58(4):363–367

190. Lord RK, Shah VA, San Filippo AN, Krishna R (2010) Novel uses of smartphones in ophthalmology. Ophthalmology 117(6). https://doi.org/10.1016/j.ophtha.2010.01.001

191. Bastawrous A (2012) Smartphone fundoscopy. Ophthalmology 119(2). https://doi.org/10.1016/j.ophtha.2011.11.014

192. Kim DY, Delori F, Mukai S (2012) Smartphone photography safety. Ophthalmology 119(10):2200–2201

193. Haddock LJ, Kim DY, Mukai S (2013) Simple, inexpensive technique for high-quality smartphone fundus photography in human and animal eyes. J Ophthalmol. https://doi.org/10.1155/2013/518479

194. Jalil M, Ferenczy SR, Shields CL (2017) iPhone 4s and iPhone 5s imaging of the eye. Ocul Oncol Pathol 3(1):49–55

195. Oluleye T (2014) Mobile phones for fundus photography in Ibadan, Sub Sahara Africa. Adv Ophthalmol Vis Syst 1(4):00020. https://doi.org/10.15406/aovs.2014.01.00020

196. Ademola-Popoola D, Olatunji V (2017) Retinal imaging with smartphone. Niger J Clin Pract 20(3):341–345
197. Sankaranarayanan R (2014) Screening for cancer in low-and middle-income countries. Ann Glob Health 80(5):412–417
198. Quinley KE, Gormley RH, Ratcliffe SJ, Shih T, Szep Z, Steiner A, Ramogola-Masire D, Kovarik CL (2011) Use of mobile telemedicine for cervical cancer screening. J Telemed Telecare 17(4):203–209
199. Ricard-Gauthier D, Wisniak A, Catarino R, van Rossum AF, Meyer-Hamme U, Negulescu R, Scaringella S, Jinoro J, Vassilakos P, Petignat P (2015) Use of smartphones as adjuvant tools for cervical cancer screening in low-resource settings. J Low Genit Dis 19(4):295–300
200. Parham GP, Mwanahamuntu MH, Pfaendler KS, Sahasrabuddhe VV, Myung D, Mkumba G, Kapambwe S, Mwanza B, Chibwesha C, Hicks ML (2010) eC3—a modern telecommunications matrix for cervical cancer prevention in Zambia. J Low Genit Dis 14(3). https://doi.o rg/10.1097/LGT.0b013e3181cd6d5e
201. Gallay C, Girardet A, Viviano M, Catarino R, Benski A-C, Tran PL, Ecabert C, Thiran J-P, Vassilakos P, Petignat P (2017) Cervical cancer screening in low-resource settings: a smartphone image application as an alternative to colposcopy. Int J Womens Health 9:455–461
202. FLIR® Systems (2017) FLIR ONE® PRO. http://www.flir.com/flirone/pro/. Accessed Dec 2017
203. Seal A, Bhattacharjee D, Naripuri M (2013) Thermal human face recognition for biometric security system. In: Srivastava R (ed) Research developments in biometrics and video processing techniques. IGI Global, USA
204. Cardone D, Pinti P, Merla A (2015) Thermal infrared imaging-based computational psychophysiology for psychometrics. Comput Math Method Med. https://doi.org/10.1155/201 5/984353
205. Garbey M, Sun N, Merla A, Pavlidis I (2007) Contact-free measurement of cardiac pulse based on the analysis of thermal imagery. IEEE Trans Biomed Eng 54(8):1418–1426
206. Sun N, Pavlidis I, Garbey M, Fei J (2006) Harvesting the thermal cardiac pulse signal. In: 9th International Conference on Medical Image Computing and Computer-Assisted Intervention, Copenhagen, Denmark, 1–6 October 2006
207. Bourlai T, Buddharaju P, Pavlidis I, Bass B (2009) On enhancing cardiac pulse measurements through thermal imaging. In: 9th International Conference on Information Technology and Applications in Biomedicine, Larnaca, Cyprus, 4–7 November 2009
208. Yang M, Liu Q, Turner T, Wu Y (2008) Vital sign estimation from passive thermal video. In: IEEE Conference on Computer Vision and Pattern Recognition, Anchorage, USA, 23–28 June 2008
209. Zhou Y, Tsiamyrtzis P, Lindner P, Timofeyev I, Pavlidis I (2013) Spatiotemporal smoothing as a basis for facial tissue tracking in thermal imaging. IEEE Trans Biomed Eng 60(5):1280–1289
210. Chekmenev SY, Farag AA, Essock EA (2007) Thermal imaging of the superficial temporal artery: an arterial pulse recovery model. In: IEEE Conference on Computer Vision and Pattern Recognition, Minneapolis, USA, 17–22 June 2007
211. Gault TR, Blumenthal N, Farag AA, Starr T (2010) Extraction of the superficial facial vasculature, vital signs waveforms and rates using thermal imaging. In: IEEE Computer Society Conference on Computer Vision and Pattern Recognition—Workshops, San Francisco, USA, 13–18 June 2010
212. Gault T, Farag A (2013) A fully automatic method to extract the heart rate from thermal video. In: IEEE Conference on Computer Vision and Pattern Recognition Workshops, Portland, USA, 23–28 June 2013
213. Murthy R, Pavlidis I (2006) Noncontact measurement of breathing function. IEEE Eng Med Biol Mag 25(3):57–67
214. Fei J, Pavlidis I (2007) Virtual thermistor. In: 29th Annual International Conference of the IEEE Engineering in Medicine and Biology Society, Lyon, France, 22–26 August 2007
215. Pereira CB, Yu X, Czaplik M, Blazek V, Venema B, Leonhardt S (2016) Estimation of breathing rate in thermal imaging videos: a pilot study on healthy human subjects. J Clin Monit Comput 31(6):1241–1254

216. Pereira CB, Yu X, Czaplik M, Rossaint R, Blazek V, Leonhardt S (2015) Remote monitoring of breathing dynamics using infrared thermography. Biomed Opt Express 6(11):4378–4394
217. Murthy JN, van Jaarsveld J, Fei J, Pavlidis I, Harrykissoon RI, Lucke JF, Faiz S, Castriotta RJ (2009) Thermal infrared imaging: a novel method to monitor airflow during polysomnography. Sleep 32(11):1521–1527
218. Lewis GF, Gatto RG, Porges SW (2011) A novel method for extracting respiration rate and relative tidal volume from infrared thermography. Psychophysiology 48(7):877–887
219. Jarczok MN, Kleber ME, Koenig J, Loerbroks A, Herr RM, Hoffmann K, Fischer JE, Benyamini Y, Thayer JF (2015) Investigating the associations of self-rated health: heart rate variability is more strongly associated than inflammatory and other frequently used biomarkers in a cross sectional occupational sample. PLoS ONE 10(2):e0117196. https://d oi.org/10.1371/journal.pone.0117196
220. Idler EL, Benyamini Y (1999) Community studies reporting association between self-rated health and mortality. Res Aging 21:392–401
221. Pinquart M (2001) Correlates of subjective health in older adults: a meta-analysis. Psychol Aging 16(3):414–426
222. Schmidt B, Loerbroks A, Herr RM, Wilson MG, Jarczok MN, Litaker D, Mauss D, Bosch JA, Fischer JE (2014) Associations between supportive leadership and employees self-rated health in an occupational sample. Int J Behav Med 21(5):750–756
223. Fuster V (1999) Epidemic of cardiovascular disease and stroke: the three main challenges. Circulation 99(9):1132–1137
224. Rothwell P, Coull A, Silver L, Fairhead J, Giles M, Lovelock C, Redgrave J, Bull L, Welch S, Cuthbertson F (2005) Population-based study of event-rate, incidence, case fatality, and mortality for all acute vascular events in all arterial territories (Oxford Vascular Study). Lancet 366(9499):1773–1783
225. Thayer JF, Yamamoto SS, Brosschot JF (2010) The relationship of autonomic imbalance, heart rate variability and cardiovascular disease risk factors. Int J Cardiol 141(2):122–131
226. Voss A, Heitmann A, Schroeder R, Peters A, Perz S (2012) Short-term heart rate variability—age dependence in healthy subjects. Physiol Meas 33(8):1289–1311
227. Hillebrand S, Gast KB, de Mutsert R, Swenne CA, Jukema JW, Middeldorp S, Rosendaal FR, Dekkers OM (2013) Heart rate variability and first cardiovascular event in populations without known cardiovascular disease: meta-analysis and dose–response meta-regression. Europace 15(5):742–749
228. Thompson PD (2011) The cardiovascular risks of diving. Undersea Hyperb Med 38(4):271–277
229. Bove AA (2011) The cardiovascular system and diving risk. Undersea Hyperb Med 38(4):261–269
230. Denoble P, Caruso J, de L Dear G, Pieper CF, Vann R (2008) Common causes of open-circuit recreational diving fatalities. Undersea Hyperb Med 35(6):393–406
231. Tervo T, Räty E, Sulander P, Holopainen JM, Jaakkola T, Parkkari K (2013) Sudden death at the wheel due to a disease attack. Traffic Inj Prev 14(2):138–144
232. Petch M (1998) Driving and heart disease. Eur Heart J 19(8):1165–1177
233. Fieselmann JF, Hendryx MS, Helms CM, Wakefield DS (1993) Respiratory rate predicts cardiopulmonary arrest for internal medicine inpatients. J Gen Intern Med 8(7):354–360
234. Melillo P, Izzo R, Orrico A, Scala P, Attanasio M, Mirra M, De Luca N, Pecchia L (2015) Automatic prediction of cardiovascular and cerebrovascular events using heart rate variability analysis. PLoS ONE 10(3):e0118504. https://doi.org/10.1371/journal.pone.0118504
235. Richman JS, Moorman JR (2000) Physiological time-series analysis using approximate entropy and sample entropy. Am J Physiol Heart Circ Physiol 278(6):H2039–H2049
236. Yentes JM, Hunt N, Schmid KK, Kaipust JP, McGrath D, Stergiou N (2013) The appropriate use of approximate entropy and sample entropy with short data sets. Ann Biomed Eng 41(2):349–365
237. Ji L, Li P, Li K, Wang X, Liu C (2015) Analysis of short-term heart rate and diastolic period variability using a refined fuzzy entropy method. Biomed Eng Online 14:64. https://doi.org/ 10.1186/s12938-015-0063-z

238. MedlinePlus (216) Coronary artery disease. MedlinePlus. https://medlineplus.gov/coronary arterydisease.html. Accessed Dec 2017

239. Banerjee R, Choudhury AD, Datta S, Pal A, Mandana KM (2017) Non invasive detection of coronary artery disease using PCG and PPG. In: Giokas K, Bokor L, Hopfgartner F (eds) eHealth 360°. Lecture Notes of the Institute for Computer Sciences, Social Informatics and Telecommunications Engineering, vol 181. Springer, Cham

240. Villarroel M, Guazzi A, Jorge J, Davis S, Watkinson P, Green G, Shenvi A, McCormick K, Tarassenko L (2014) Continuous non-contact vital sign monitoring in neonatal intensive care unit. Healthc Technol Lett 1(3):87–91

241. Werth J, Atallah L, Andriessen P, Long X, Zwartkruis-Pelgrim E, Aarts RM (2017) Unobtrusive sleep state measurements in preterm infants—a review. Sleep Med Rev 32:109–122

242. Soto RG, Fu ES, Vila H Jr, Miguel RV (2004) Capnography accurately detects apnea during monitored anesthesia care. Anesth Analg 99(2):379–382

243. Berry R (2002) Esophageal and nasal pressure monitoring during sleep. In: Sateia M, Carskadon MA, Lee-Chiong TL (eds) Sleep medicine. Hanley & Belfus, USA

244. Berry RB, Brooks R, Gamaldo CE, Harding SM, Marcus C, Vaughn B (2012) The AASM manual for the scoring of sleep and associated events: Rules, terminology and technical specifications. In: American Academy of Sleep Medicine. Available via https://aasm.org/cl inical-resources/scoring-manual/. Accessed Mar 2018

245. Bornstein SK (1982) Respiratory monitoring during sleep: polysomnography. In: Guilleminault C (ed) Sleeping and waking disorders: indications and techniques. Addison-Wesley Publishing Company, USA

246. Lee-Chiong TL (2003) Monitoring respiration during sleep. Clin Chest Med 24(2):297–306. https://doi.org/10.1016/S0272-5231(03)00021-2

247. Richter DW (2003) Commentary on eupneic breathing patterns and gasping. Respir Physiol Neurobiol 139(1):121–130

248. Wilburta LQ, Pooler M, Tamparo CD, Dahl BM, Morris J (2013) Delmar's comprehensive medical assisting: administrative and clinical competencies. Cengage Learning, USA

249. White GC (2012) Basic clinical lab competencies for respiratory care: an integrated approach. Cengage Learning, USA

250. Tufik S, Santos-Silva R, Taddei JA, Bittencourt LRA (2010) Obstructive sleep apnea syndrome in the Sao Paulo epidemiologic sleep study. Sleep Med 11(5):441–446

251. Heinzer R, Vat S, Marques-Vidal P, Marti-Soler H, Andries D, Tobback N, Mooser V, Preisig M, Malhotra A, Waeber G (2015) Prevalence of sleep-disordered breathing in the general population: the HypnoLaus study. Lancet Respir Med 3(4):310–318

252. Peppard PE, Young T, Barnet JH, Palta M, Hagen EW, Hla KM (2013) Increased prevalence of sleep-disordered breathing in adults. Am J Epidemiol 177(9):1006–1014

253. Ott SR, Korostovtseva L, Schmidt M, Horvath T, Brill A-K, Bassetti CL (2017) Sleep-disordered breathing: clinical features, pathophysiology and diagnosis. Swiss Med Wkly 147:w14436. https://doi.org/10.4414/smw.2017.14436

254. Franklin KA, Lindberg E (2015) Obstructive sleep apnea is a common disorder in the population—a review on the epidemiology of sleep apnea. J Thorac Dis 7(8):1311–1322

255. Ryan CM, Wilton K, Bradley TD, Alshaer H (2017) In-hospital diagnosis of sleep apnea in stroke patients using a portable acoustic device. Sleep Breath 21(2):453–460

256. Johnson KG, Johnson DC (2010) Frequency of sleep apnea in stroke and TIA patients: a meta-analysis. J Clin Sleep Med 6(2):131–137

257. Hermann DM, Siccoli M, Kirov P, Gugger M, Bassetti CL (2007) Central periodic breathing during sleep in acute ischemic stroke. Stroke 38(3):1082–1084

258. Nopmaneejumruslers C, Kaneko Y, Hajek V, Zivanovic V, Bradley TD (2005) Cheyne-Stokes respiration in stroke: relationship to hypocapnia and occult cardiac dysfunction. Am J Respir Crit Care Med 171(9):1048–1052

259. Alshaer H, Levchenko A, Bradley TD, Pong S, Tseng W-H, Fernie GR (2013) A system for portable sleep apnea diagnosis using an embedded data capturing module. J Clin Monit Comput 27(3):303–311

260. Masa JF, Duran-Cantolla J, Capote F, Cabello M, Abad J, Garcia-Rio F, Ferrer A, Mayos M, Gonzalez-Mangado N, de la Peña M (2014) Effectiveness of home single-channel nasal pressure for sleep apnea diagnosis. Sleep 37(12):1953–1961

261. Guilleminault C, Peraita R, Souquet M, Dement WC (1975) Apneas during sleep in infants: possible relationship with sudden infant death syndrome. Science 190(4215):677–679

262. Alekhin M, Anishchenko L, Zhuravlev A, Ivashov S, Korostovtseva L, Sviryaev Y, Konradi A, Parashin V, Bogomolov A (2013) Estimation of information value of diagnostic data obtained by bioradiolocation pneumography in non-contact screening of sleep apnea syndrome. Biomed Eng. https://doi.org/10.1007/s10527-013-9343-8

263. Isidoro SI, Salvaggio A, Bue AL, Romano S, Marrone O, Insalaco G (2015) Effect of obstructive sleep apnea diagnosis on health related quality of life. Health Qual Life Outcomes 13:68. https://doi.org/10.1186/s12955-015-0253-1

264. Stewart SA, Skomro R, Reid J, Penz E, Fenton M, Gjevre J, Cotton D (2015) improvement in obstructive sleep apnea diagnosis and management wait times: a retrospective analysis of a home management pathway for obstructive sleep apnea. Can Respir J 22(3):167–170

265. Kim RD, Kapur VK, Redline-Bruch J, Rueschman M, Auckley DH, Benca RM, Foldvary-Schafer NR, Iber C, Zee PC, Rosen CL (2015) An economic evaluation of home versus laboratory-based diagnosis of obstructive sleep apnea. Sleep 38(7):1027–1037

266. Young T, Palta M, Dempsey J, Peppard PE, Nieto FJ, Hla KM (2009) Burden of sleep apnea: rationale, design, and major findings of the Wisconsin Sleep Cohort study. WMJ 108(5):246–249

267. Lorenzi-Filho G, Genta P, Drager L (2017) Are we missing obstructive sleep apnea diagnosis? Rev Port Pneumol 23(2):55–56

268. Taplidou SA, Hadjileontiadis LJ (2007) Wheeze detection based on time-frequency analysis of breath sounds. Comput Biol Med 37(8):1073–1083

269. Brooks D, Thomas J (1995) Interrater reliability of auscultation of breath sounds among physical therapists. Phys Ther 75(12):1082–1088

270. Spiteri M, Cook D, Clarke S (1988) Reliability of eliciting physical signs in examination of the chest. Lancet 331(8590):873–875

271. Prodhan P, Rosa RSD, Shubina M, Haver KE, Matthews BD, Buck S, Kacmarek RM, Noviski NN (2008) Wheeze detection in the pediatric intensive care unit: comparison among physician, nurses, respiratory therapists, and a computerized respiratory sound monitor. Respir Care 53(10):1304–1309

272. Kandaswamy A, Kumar CS, Ramanathan RP, Jayaraman S, Malmurugan N (2004) Neural classification of lung sounds using wavelet coefficients. Comput Biol Med 34(6):523–537

273. Sengupta N, Sahidullah M, Saha G (2016) Lung sound classification using cepstral-based statistical features. Comput Biol Med 75:118–129

274. Abbas A, Fahim A (2010) An automated computerized auscultation and diagnostic system for pulmonary diseases. J Med Syst 34(6):1149–1155

275. Yamashita M, Matsunaga S, Miyahara S (2011) Discrimination between healthy subjects and patients with pulmonary emphysema by detection of abnormal respiration. In: IEEE International Conference on Acoustics, Speech and Signal Processing, Prague, Czech Republic, 22–27 May 2011

276. Datta S, Choudhury AD, Deshpande P, Bhattacharya S, Pal A (2017) Automated lung sound analysis for detecting pulmonary abnormalities. In: 39th Annual International Conference of the IEEE Engineering in Medicine and Biology Society, Seogwipo, South Korea, 11–15 July 2017

277. Kevat AC, Kalirajah A, Roseby R (2017) Digital stethoscopes compared to standard auscultation for detecting abnormal paediatric breath sounds. Eur J Pediatr 176(7):989–992

278. Chamberlain D, Kodgule R, Ganelin D, Miglani V, Fletcher RR (2016) Application of semi-supervised deep learning to lung sound analysis. In: 38th Annual International Conference of the IEEE Engineering in Medicine and Biology Society, Orlando, USA, 16–20 August 2016

279. Marciniuk D, Ferkol T, Nana A, de Oca MM, Rabe K, Billo N, Zar H (2014) Respiratory diseases in the world. Realities of today—opportunities for tomorrow. In: Afr J Respir Med.

Available via: https://pdfs.semanticscholar.org/df52/2102c7d0e3334093c394be1e668d7174 7221.pdf. Accessed Mar 2018

280. Gruffydd-Jones K, Nicholson I, Best L, Connell E (1999) Why don't patients attend the asthma clinic? Prim Care Resp J 7:36–38

281. Royal College of Physicians (2015) Why asthma still kills: The National Review of Asthma Deaths (NRAD) confidential enquiry report. London, RCP, 2014. www.rcplondon.ac.uk/sit es/default/files/why-asthma-still-kills-full-report.pdf. Accessed Mar 2018

282. Pinnock H, Slack R, Pagliari C, Price D, Sheikh A (2007) Understanding the potential role of mobile phone-based monitoring on asthma self-management: qualitative study. Clin Exp Allergy 37(5):794–802

283. Mohammadi D (2018) Smart inhalers: will they help to improve asthma care? Pharm J—A Royal Pharmaceutical Society Publication. Available via: https://www.pharmaceutical-jour nal.com/news-and-analysis/features/smart-inhalers-will-they-help-to-improve-asthma-care/ 20202556.article. Accessed Mar 2018

284. Thuemmler C, Bai C (2017) Health 4.0: application of industry 4.0 design principles in future asthma management. In: Health 4.0: how virtualization and big data are revolutionizing healthcare. Springer

285. Son J, Brennan PF, Zhou S (2016) Rescue inhaler usage prediction in smart asthma management systems using joint mixed effects logistic regression model. IIE Trans 48(4):333–346

286. Heaney LG, McGarvey LP (2017) Personalised medicine for asthma and chronic obstructive pulmonary disease. Respiration 93(3):153–161

287. Wiecha JM, Adams WG, Rybin D, Rizzodepaoli M, Keller J, Clay JM (2015) Evaluation of a web-based asthma self-management system: a randomised controlled pilot trial. BMC Pulm Med 15:17. https://doi.org/10.1186/s12890-015-0007-1

288. Burbank AJ, Lewis SD, Hewes M, Schellhase DE, Rettiganti M, Hall-Barrow J, Bylander LA, Brown RH, Perry TT (2015) Mobile-based asthma action plans for adolescents. J Asthma 52(6):583–586

289. Thomson J, Hass C, Horn I, Kleine E, Mitchell S, Gary K, Ahmed I, Hamel D, Amresh A (2017) Aspira: employing a serious game in an mHealth app to improve asthma outcomes. In: IEEE 5th International Conference on Serious Games and Applications for Health, Perth, Australia, 2–4 April 2017

290. Al-Dowaihi D, Al-Ajlan M, Al-Zahrani N, Al-Quwayfili N, al-Jwiser N, Kanjo E (2013) Mbreath: asthma monitoring system on the go. In: International Conference on Computer Medical Applications, Sousse, Tunisia, 20–22 January 2013

291. Negar N (2015) Towards mHealth solutions for asthma patients. Dissertation, Marquette University

292. WHO WH (1996) The global burden of disease: a comprehensive assessment of mortality and disability from diseases, injuries, and risk factors in 1990 and projected to 2020: summary. http://apps.who.int/iris/bitstream/handle/10665/41864/0965546608_eng.pdf;jsessionid=47B 0730D84595AFC9A512D602E51E10E?sequence=1. Accessed Mar 2018

293. Kessler RC, Greenberg PE (2002) The economic burden of anxiety and stress disorders. In: Davis KL, American College of Neurophsychopharmacology (eds) Neuropsychopharmacology: the fifth generation of progress. Lippincott Williams & Wilkins, Pennsylvania

294. Yerkes RM, Dodson J (1968) The relation of strength of stimulus to rapidity of habit-formation. In: Punishment: Issues and experiments. J Comp Neurol Psychol. https://doi.org/ 10.1002/cne.920180503

295. Cohen S (1980) Aftereffects of stress on human performance and social behavior: a review of research and theory. Psychol Bull 88(1):82–108

296. Schuler RS (1980) Definition and conceptualization of stress in organizations. Organ Behav Hum Perform 25(2):184–215

297. Kalia M (2002) Assessing the economic impact of stress—the modern day hidden epidemic. Metabolism 51(6 Suppl 1):49–53

298. WHO (2008) The global burden of disease: 2004 update. http://www.who.int/healthinfo/gl obal_burden_disease/2004_report_update/en/. Accessed Mar 2018

299. Arnsten AF (2015) Stress weakens prefrontal networks: molecular insults to higher cognition. Nat Neurosci 18(10):1376–1385
300. Rowden P, Matthews G, Watson B, Biggs H (2011) The relative impact of work-related stress, life stress and driving environment stress on driving outcomes. Accid Anal Prev 43(4):1332–1340
301. Ge Y, Qu W, Jiang C, Du F, Sun X, Zhang K (2014) The effect of stress and personality on dangerous driving behavior among Chinese drivers. Accid Anal Prev 73:34–40
302. Hill JD, Boyle LN (2007) Driver stress as influenced by driving maneuvers and roadway conditions. Transp Res Part F Traffic Psychol Behav 10(3):177–186
303. The American Institute of Stress (2011) Workplace stress. https://www.stress.org/workplac e-stress/. Accessed Mar 2018
304. Pavlidis I, Dowdall J, Sun N, Puri C, Fei J, Garbey M (2007) Interacting with human physiology. Comput Vis Image Underst 108(1):150–170
305. Engert V, Merla A, Grant JA, Cardone D, Tusche A, Singer T (2014) Exploring the use of thermal infrared imaging in human stress research. PLoS ONE 9(3):e90782
306. Cardone D, Merla A (2017) New frontiers for applications of thermal infrared imaging devices: computational psychopshysiology in the neurosciences. Sensors 17(5):1042. https:// doi.org/10.3390/s17051042
307. Thayer JF, Åhs F, Fredrikson M, Sollers JJ, Wager TD (2012) A meta-analysis of heart rate variability and neuroimaging studies: implications for heart rate variability as a marker of stress and health. Neurosci Biobehav Rev 36(2):747–756
308. Motomura N, Sakurai A, Yotsuya Y (2001) Reduction of mental stress with lavender odorant. Percept Motor Skill 93(3):713–718
309. Tillotson J eScent®. Sensory Design & Technology Ltd. http://www.escent.ai/. Accessed Nov 2017
310. Byrom B (2015) Brain monitoring devices in clinical trials. Appl Clin Trials. http://www.a ppliedclinicaltrialsonline.com/brain-monitoring-devices-clinical-trials. Accessed Mar 2018
311. Poltavski DV (2015) The use of single-electrode wireless EEG in biobehavioral investi-gations. In: Rasooly A, Herold K (eds) Mobile health technologies. Methods in molecular biology, vol 1256. Humana Press, New York
312. Rodriguez Ortega A, Rey Solaz B, Raya A, Luis M (2013) Validation of a low-cost EEG device for mood induction studies. Stud Health Technol Inform 191:43–47
313. Ring E, Collins A, Bacon P, Cosh J (1974) Quantitation of thermography in arthritis using multi-isothermal analysis. II. Effect of nonsteroidal anti-inflammatory therapy on the thermographic index. Ann Rheum Dis 33(4):353–356
314. Collins A, Ring E, Cosh J, Bacon P (1974) Quantitation of thermography in arthritis using multi-isothermal analysis. I. The thermographic index. Ann Rheum Dis 33(2):113–115
315. Bacon P, Ring E, Collins A (1977) Thermography in the assessment of anti-rheumatic agents. In: Gordon JL, Hazleman BL (eds) Rheumatoid arthritis. Elsevler, Amsterdam
316. Handwerker H (1990) Assessment of the effect of ibuprofen and other non-steroidal anti-rheumatic drugs in experimental algesimetry. Z Rheumatol 50(Suppl 1):15–18
317. Bruning RS, Dahmus JD, Kenney WL, Holowatz LA (2013) Aspirin and clopidogrel alter core temperature and skin blood flow during heat stress. Med Sci Sport Exer 45(4):674–682
318. Hughes JH, Henry RE, Daly MJ (1984) Influence of ethanol and ambient temperature on skin blood flow. Ann Emerg Med 13(8):597–600
319. Wolf R, Tüzün B, Tüzün Y (1999) Alcohol ingestion and the cutaneous vasculature. Clin Dermatol 17(4):395–403
320. Ammer K, Melnizky P, Rathkolb O (2003) Skin temperature after intake of sparkling wine, still wine or sparkling water. Thermol Int 13(3):99–102
321. Mannara G, Salvatori G, Pizzuti G (1993) Ethyl alcohol induced skin temperature changes evaluated by thermography. Preliminary results. Boll Soc Ital Biol Sper 69(10):587–594
322. Morley JE (2015) Dehydration, hypernatremia, and hyponatremia. Clin Geriatr Med 31(3):389–399

323. Stookey JD (2005) High prevalence of plasma hypertonicity among community-dwelling older adults: results from NHANES III. J Am Diet Assoc 105(8):1231–1239

324. Frangeskou M, Lopez-Valcarcel B, Serra-Majem L (2015) Dehydration in the elderly: a review focused on economic burden. J Nutr Health Aging 19(6):619–627

325. Pash E, Parikh N, Hashemi L (2014) Economic burden associated with hospital postadmission dehydration. Jpen J Parenter Enteral Nutr 38(2 suppl):58S–64S

326. Hooper L, Bunn D, Jimoh FO, Fairweather-Tait SJ (2014) Water-loss dehydration and aging. Mech Ageing Dev 136:50–58

327. Serra-Majem L (2015) Opening remarks: the burden of disease attributable to hydration in Europe. Nutr Hosp 32(2):3

328. Clarys P, Alewaeters K, Lambrecht R, Barel A (2000) Skin color measurements: comparison between three instruments: the Chromameter®, the DermaSpectrometer® and the Mexameter®. Skin Res Technol 6(4):230–238

329. Konica Minolta (2015) Color measurement. http://sensing.konicaminolta.asia/applications/color-measurement/. Accessed Feb 2016

330. Daniel LC, Heckman CJ, Kloss JD, Manne SL (2009) Comparing alternative methods of measuring skin color and damage. Cancer Causes Control 20(3):313–321

331. Yaroslavsky I, Childs J, Altshuler GB, Zenzie HH, Cohen R (2012) Objective measurement device for melanin optical density: dosimetry for laser and ipls in aesthetic treatments. http://bramptonlaserclinic.com/pdf/skintel_technical.pdf. Accessed Dec 2017

332. Macdonald HM, Mavroeidi A, Aucott LA, Diffey BL, Fraser WD, Ormerod AD, Reid DM (2011) Skin color change in Caucasian postmenopausal women predicts summer-winter change in 25-hydroxyvitamin D: findings from the ANSAViD cohort study. J Clin Endocr Metab 96(6):1677–1686

333. Zvornicanin E, Zvornicanin J, Hadziefendic B (2014) The use of smart phones in ophthalmology. Acta Inform Med 22(3):206–209

334. Bastawrous A, Cheeseman R, Kumar A (2012) iPhones for eye surgeons. Eye 26(3):343–354

335. Lakshminarayanan V, Zelek J, McBride A (2015) "Smartphone science" in eye care and medicine. Opt Photonics News 26(1):44–51

336. Cheng NM, Chakrabarti R, Kam JK (2014) iPhone applications for eye care professionals: a review of current capabilities and concerns. Telemed e-Health 20(4):385–387

337. Rodríguez-Vallejo M (2016) Comment on: 'effectiveness of a smartphone application for testing near-visual acuity'. Eye 30(6):898–899

338. Pathipati AS, Wood EH, Lam CK, Sáles CS, Moshfeghi DM (2016) Visual acuity measured with a smartphone app is more accurate than Snellen testing by emergency department providers. Graefes Arch Clinl Exp Ophthalmol 254(6):1175–1180

339. Tofigh S, Shortridge E, Elkeeb A, Godley B (2015) Effectiveness of a smartphone application for testing near visual acuity. Eye 29(11):1464–1468

340. Yau JW, Rogers SL, Kawasaki R, Lamoureux EL, Kowalski JW, Bek T, Chen S-J, Dekker JM, Fletcher A, Grauslund J (2012) Global prevalence and major risk factors of diabetic retinopathy. Diabetes Care 35(3):556–564

341. Viswanath K, McGavin DM (2003) Diabetic retinopathy: clinical findings and management. Community Eye Health 16(46):21–24

342. Willis JR, Doan QV, Gleeson M, Haskova Z, Ramulu P, Morse L, Cantrell RA (2017) Vision-related functional burden of diabetic retinopathy across severity levels in the United States. JAMA Ophthalmol 135(9):926–932

343. Vashist P, Singh S, Gupta N, Saxena R (2011) Role of early screening for diabetic retinopathy in patients with diabetes mellitus: an overview. Indian J Community Med 36(4):247–252

344. Rajalakshmi R, Amutha A, Ranjani H, Ali MK, Unnikrishnan R, Anjana RM, Narayan KV, Mohan V (2014) Prevalence and risk factors for diabetic retinopathy in Asian Indians with young onset type 1 and type 2 diabetes. J Diabetes Complications 28(3):291–297

345. Micheletti JM, Hendrick AM, Khan FN, Ziemer DC, Pasquel FJ (2016) Current and next generation portable screening devices for diabetic retinopathy. J Diabetes Sci Technol 10(2):295–300

346. Optical V Pictor Plus—digital ophtalmic imager (2017) http://volk.com/pictorplus/. Accessed Dec 2017
347. iExaminer Welch Allyn (2017) https://www.welchallyn.com. Accessed Dec 2017
348. Pérez GM, Swart W, Munyenyembe JK, Saranchuk P (2014) Barriers to pilot mobile teleophthalmology in a rural hospital in Southern Malawi. Pan Afr Med J 19:136. https://doi.org/10.11604/pamj.2014.19.136.5196
349. Toy BC, Myung DJ, He L, Pan CK, Chang RT, Polkinhorne A, Merrell D, Foster D, Blumenkranz MS (2016) Smartphone-based dilated fundus photography and near visual acuity testing as inexpensive screening tools to detect referral warranted diabetic eye disease. Retina 36(5):1000–1008
350. Myung D, Jais A, He L, Blumenkranz MS, Chang RT (2014) 3D printed smartphone indirect lens adapter for rapid, high quality retinal imaging. J Mob Technol Med 3(1):9–15
351. Brackbill RM, Thorpe LE, DiGrande L, Perrin M, Sapp JH, Wu D, Campolucci S, Walker DJ, Cone J, Pulliam P (2006) Surveillance for World Trade Center disaster health effects among survivors of collapsed and damaged buildings. MMWR Surveill Summ 55(2):1–18
352. Mines M, Thach A, Mallonee S, Hildebrand L, Shariat S (2000) Ocular injuries sustained by survivors of the Oklahoma City bombing. Ophthalmology 107(5):837–843
353. WHO (2012) Cervical cancer: estimated incidence, mortality and prevalence worldwide in 2012. http://globocan.iarc.fr/old/FactSheets/cancers/cervix-new.asp. Accessed Dec 2017
354. Forman D, de Martel C, Lacey CJ, Soerjomataram I, Lortet-Tieulent J, Bruni L, Vignat J, Ferlay J, Bray F, Plummer M (2012) Global burden of human papillomavirus and related diseases. Vaccine 30:F12–F23
355. WHO (2014) CI5PLUS: cancer incidence in five continents time trends. http://ci5.iarc.fr/CI5plus/Default.aspx. Accessed Dec 2017
356. American Cancer Society (2017) Global burden of cancer in women: current status, trends, and interventions. https://www.cancer.org/content/dam/cancer-org/research/cancer-facts-and-statistics/global-cancer-facts-and-figures/global-burden-of-cancer-in-women.pdf. Accessed Mar 2018
357. Technologies MOD reach every patient. http://www.mobileodt.com/. Accessed Dec 2017
358. International Agency for Research on Cancer (2011) Recent evidence on cervical cancer screening in low-resource settings. http://screening.iarc.fr/doc/ACCP_cxca_screening_2011.pdf. Accessed Mar 2018
359. Wright TC, Kuhn L (2012) Alternative approaches to cervical cancer screening for developing countries. Best Pract Res Clin Obstet Gynaecol 26(2):197–208
360. Arbyn M, Sankaranarayanan R, Muwonge R, Keita N, Dolo A, Mbalawa CG, Nouhou H, Sakande B, Wesley R, Somanathan T (2008) Pooled analysis of the accuracy of five cervical cancer screening tests assessed in eleven studies in Africa and India. Int J Cancer 123(1):153–160
361. Cronjé HS, Parham GP, Cooreman BF, De Beer A, Divall P, Bam RH (2003) A comparison of four screening methods for cervical neoplasia in a developing country. Am J Obstet Gynecol 188(2):395–400
362. Stafl A (1981) Cervicography: a new method for cervical cancer detection. Am J Obstet Gynecol 139(7):815–821
363. De Vuyst H, Claeys P, Njiru S, Muchiri L, Steyaert S, De Sutter P, Van Marck E, Bwayo J, Temmerman M (2005) Comparison of pap smear, visual inspection with acetic acid, human papillomavirus DNA-PCR testing and cervicography. Int J Gynecol Obstet 89(2):120–126
364. Bomfim-Hyppólito S, Santana Franco E, de Matos Gomes, Meneses Franco R, Matos de Albuquerque C, Nunes G (2006) Cervicography as an adjunctive test to visual inspection with acetic acid in cervical cancer detection screening. Int J Gynecol Obstet 92(1):58–63
365. Pretorius RG, Bao YP, Belinson JL, Burchette RJ, Smith JS, Qiao YL (2007) Inappropriate gold standard bias in cervical cancer screening studies. Int J Cancer 121(10):2218–2224
366. Urner E, Delavy M, Catarino R, Viviano M, Meyer-Hamme U, Benski A-C, Jinoro J, Heriniainasolo JL, Undurraga M, De Vuyst H (2017) A smartphone-based approach for triage of human papillomavirus-positive sub-Saharan African women: a prospective study. JMIR mHealth uHealth 5(5):e72

367. Ng SC, Shi HY, Hamidi N, Underwood FE, Tang W, Benchimol EI, Panaccione R, Ghosh S, Wu JC, Chan FK (2017) Worldwide incidence and prevalence of inflammatory bowel disease in the 21st century: a systematic review of population-based studies. Lancet 390(10114):2769–2778

368. Dionisio PM, Gurudu SR, Leighton JA, Leontiadis GI, Fleischer DE, Hara AK, Heigh RI, Shiff AD, Sharma VK (2010) Capsule endoscopy has a significantly higher diagnostic yield in patients with suspected and established small-bowel Crohn's disease: a meta-analysis. Am J Gastroenterol 105(6):1240–1248

369. Mow WS, Lo SK, Targan SR, Dubinsky MC, Treyzon L, Abreu-Martin MT, Papadakis KA, Vasiliauskas EA (2004) Initial experience with wireless capsule enteroscopy in the diagnosis and management of inflammatory bowel disease. Clin Gastroenterol Hepatol 2(1):31–40

370. Swain P, Fritscher-Ravens A (2004) Role of video endoscopy in managing small bowel disease. Gut 53(12):1866–1875

371. Flamant M, Trang C, Maillard O, Sacher-Huvelin S, Le Rhun M, Galmiche J-P, Bourreille A (2013) The prevalence and outcome of jejunal lesions visualized by small bowel capsule endoscopy in Crohn's disease. Inflamm Bowel Dis 19(7):1390–1396

372. Ilangovan R, Burling D, George A, Gupta A, Marshall M, Taylor S (2012) CT enterography: review of technique and practical tips. Br J Radiol 85(1015):876–886

373. Jaffe TA, Gaca AM, Delaney S, Yoshizumi TT, Toncheva G, Nguyen G, Frush DP (2007) Radiation doses from small-bowel follow-through and abdominopelvic MDCT in Crohn's disease. Am J Roentgenol 189(5):1015–1022

374. Dignass A, Van Assche G, Lindsay J, Lémann M, Söderholm J, Colombel J, Danese S, D'Hoore A, Gassull M, Gomollón F (2010) The second European evidence-based consensus on the diagnosis and management of Crohn's disease: current management. J Crohn's Colitis 4(1):28–62

375. Jensen MD, Nathan T, Rafaelsen SR, Kjeldsen J (2011) Diagnostic accuracy of capsule endoscopy for small bowel Crohn's disease is superior to that of MR enterography or CT enterography. Clin Gastroenterol Hepatol 9(2):124–129

376. Leighton JA, Gralnek IM, Cohen SA, Toth E, Cave DR, Wolf DC, Mullin GE, Ketover SR, Legnani PE, Seidman EG (2014) Capsule endoscopy is superior to small-bowel follow-through and equivalent to ileocolonoscopy in suspected Crohn's disease. Clin Gastroenterol Hepatol 12(4):609–615

377. Ho IK, Cash BD, Cohen H, Hanauer SB, Inkster M, Johnson DA, Maher MM, Rex DK, Saad A, Singh A (2014) Radiation exposure in gastroenterology: improving patient and staff protection. Am J Gastroenterol 109(8):1180–1194

378. Allez M, Lemann M, Bonnet J, Cattan P, Jian R, Modigliani R (2002) Long term outcome of patients with active Crohn's disease exhibiting extensive and deep ulcerations at colonoscopy1. Am J Gastroenterol 97(4):947–953

379. Baert F, Moortgat L, Van Assche G, Caenepeel P, Vergauwe P, De Vos M, Stokkers P, Hommes D, Rutgeerts P, Vermeire S (2010) Mucosal healing predicts sustained clinical remission in patients with early-stage Crohn's disease. Gastroenterology 138(2):463–468

380. Kopylov U, Yablecovitch D, Lahat A, Neuman S, Levhar N, Greener T, Klang E, Rozendorn N, Amitai MM, Ben-Horin S (2015) Detection of small bowel mucosal healing and deep remission in patients with known small bowel Crohn's disease using biomarkers, capsule endoscopy, and imaging. Am J Gastroenterol 110(9):1316–1323

381. Phillips CJ (2006) Economic burden of chronic pain. Expert Rev Pharmacoecon Outcomes Res 6(5):591–601

382. Williams C (2015) Pain drain: the economic and social costs of chronic pain. https://theco nversation.com/pain-drain-the-economic-and-social-costs-of-chronic-pain-49666. Accessed Mar 2018

383. Simon LS (2012) Relieving pain in America: a blueprint for transforming prevention, care, education, and research. J Pain Palliat Care Pharmacother 26(2):197–198

384. Breivik H, Eisenberg E, O'Brien T (2013) The individual and societal burden of chronic pain in Europe: the case for strategic prioritisation and action to improve knowledge and availability of appropriate care. BMC Public Hhealth 13:1229. https://doi.org/10.1186/1471-2458-13-1229

385. Prichep LS, John ER, Howard B, Merkin H, Hiesiger EM (2011) Evaluation of the pain matrix using EEG source localization: a feasibility study. Pain Med 12(8):1241–1248
386. dos Santos Pinheiro ES, de Queirós FC, Montoya P, Santos CL, do Nascimento MA, Ito CH, Silva M, Santos DBN, Benevides S, Miranda JGV (2016) Electroencephalographic patterns in chronic pain: a systematic review of the literature. PLoS One 11(2):e0149085
387. PainQx (2018) Objective pain measurement. https://www.painqx.com/about-us. Accessed Mar 2018
388. Waber RL, Shiv B, Carmon Z, Ariely D (2008) Commercial features of placebo and therapeutic. JAMA 299(9):1016–1017
389. Krauth C, Bartling T (2017) Lohnt sich Rehabilitation? Bundesgesundheitsblatt-Gesundheitsforschung-Gesundheitsschutz 60(4):394–401
390. Jitaree S, Phinyomark A, Hu H, Phukpattaranont P, Limsakul C (2012) Design of EMG biofeedback system for lower-limb exercises of the elderly using video games. J Sports Sci Health 13(2):S175–S187
391. Kim K, Kang J, Lee Y, Moon C, Choi H, Mun C (2011) The development of muscle training system using the electromyogram and interactive game for physical rehabilitation. In: International Conference on Biomedical Engineering, Kuala Lumpur, Malaysia, 20–23 June 2011
392. Lyons G, Sharma P, Baker M, O'Malley S, Shanahan A (2003) A computer game-based EMG biofeedback system for muscle rehabilitation. In: Annual International Conference of the IEEE Engineering in Medicine and Biology Society, Cancun, Mexico, 17–21 September 2003
393. Reyes HC, Arteaga JM (2016) Multidisciplinary production of interactive environments to support occupational therapies. J Biomed Inform 63:90–99
394. Reyes HC, Arteaga JM (2018) Occupational therapy for people with physical disability using interactive environments. Universal Access Inf Soc 17(1):67–81
395. Joshi CD, Lahiri U, Thakor NV (2013) Classification of gait phases from lower limb EMG: application to exoskeleton orthosis. In: Point-of-Care Healthcare Technologies, Bangalore, India, 16–18 January 2013
396. Cavallaro EE, Rosen J, Perry JC, Burns S (2006) Real-time myoprocessors for a neural controlled powered exoskeleton arm. IEEE Trans Biomed Eng 53(11):2387–2396
397. Kiguchi K, Kariya S, Watanabe K, Izumi K, Fukuda T (2001) An exoskeletal robot for human elbow motion support-sensor fusion, adaptation, and control. IEEE Trans Syst Man Cybern B Cybern 31(3):353–361
398. Rosen J, Fuchs MB, Arcan M (1999) Performances of Hill-type and neural network muscle models—toward a myosignal-based exoskeleton. Comput Biomed Res 32(5):415–439
399. Song R, Tong K (2005) Using recurrent artificial neural network model to estimate voluntary elbow torque in dynamic situations. Med Biol Eng Comput 43(4):473–480
400. Lenzi T, De Rossi SMM, Vitiello N, Carrozza MC (2012) Intention-based EMG control for powered exoskeletons. IEEE Trans Biomed Eng 59(8):2180–2190

Printed in the United States
By Bookmasters